CranioSacral
THERAPY

Touchstone for Natural Healing

John E. Upledger, DO, OMM

North Atlantic Books
Berkeley, California

UI Enterprises
Palm Beach Gardens, Florida

Published by
North Atlantic Books
P O Box 12327, Berkeley, California 94712

UI Enterprises
11211 Prosperity Farms Road, Palm Beach Gardens, Florida 33410

Front cover design © 2001 Carolina de Bartolo.
Printed in the United States of America.

CranioSacral Therapy: Touchstone for Natural Healing is sponsored by the Society for the Study of Native Arts and Sciences, a nonprofit educational corporation whose goals are to develop an educational and crosscultural perspective linking various scientific, social, and artistic fields; to nurture a holistic view of arts, sciences, humanities, and healing; and to publish and distribute literature on the relationship of mind, body, and nature.

North Atlantic Books' publications are available through most bookstores. For further information, call 800-337-2665 or visit our website at www.northatlanticbooks.com.

Substantial discounts on bulk quantities are available to corporations, professional associations, and other organizations. For details and discount information, contact our special sales department.

Library of Congress Cataloging-in-Publication Data
Upledger, John E., 1932–
   CranioSacral Therapy: Touchstone for Natural Healing / John E. Upledger
      p. cm.
   ISBN 1-55643-368-9 (trade paper : alk. paper)
      1. Craniosacral therapy. I. Title.
   RZ399.C73.U655 2000
   615.8'2--dc21   00-045247
                                          CIP

   4 5 6 7 8 9 / 09 08 07 06 05

CranioSacral
THERAPY

Touchstone for Natural Healing

Contents

Important Note

Medical knowledge is ever changing. As new research and clinical experiences broaden our knowledge, changes in treatment and drug therapy may be required. The authors and editors of the material herein have consulted sources believed to be reliable in their efforts to provide information that is complete and in accordance with the standards accepted at the time of publication.

However, the authors, editors, publisher, or any other party who has been involved in the preparation of this work, do not warrant the information contained herein and are not responsible for any errors or omissions resulting from use of such information.

Readers are encouraged to confirm the information contained herein with other sources to best suit their particular situations.

Some of the product names, patents and registered designs referred to in this book are in fact registered trademarks or proprietary names, even though specific reference to this fact is not always made in the text. Therefore, the appearance of a name without designation as proprietary is not to be construed as a representation by the publisher that it is in the public domain.

1

The Craniosacral System

What It Is and How We Found It

To know what CranioSacral Therapy is for you it is important that you have some understanding of the *craniosacral system* and what it does. The *craniosacral system* probably exists in all living things that have a spine, although its presence has not in fact been confirmed in many creatures called *"vertebrates."*

My own experience with what later came to be named the *craniosacral system* began in 1971. I was assisting a neurosurgeon with the removal of a calcium plaque. This plaque was about the size of a dime. It had formed upon the outer surface of the *meningeal membrane system*.

The *meningeal system* envelops the whole brain and *spinal cord* in each of us. It is composed of three layers of membrane. The outermost layer is called the *"dura mater."* It is tough and waterproof. Without it there would be no *craniosacral system*. The innermost layer is called the *"pia mater."* This layer follows every contour and groove of the brain and *spinal cord*. It maintains surface contact with them and carries blood vessels that service the brain and *spinal cord*. The middle layer of the *meningeal system* is called the *arachnoid membrane*. It serves as a gliding surface between the outer and inner layers of *meningeal membrane*. There is fluid, called *"cerebrospinal fluid,"* between each of the three layers of membrane of the *meningeal system*. This fluid, among other things we will discuss a little later, serves as a lubricant between these layers of *meningeal membrane* as they move in relation to each other. If these layers stick together in an area, the result is pain. Where the pain locates depends upon where the membranes are stuck together and whether or not nerves are involved or "pinched" in the stuck areas. Pain can be local or referred to a distance. It is the job of the CranioSacral Therapist to identify areas where membranes are not free to glide and thus are sources of pain in distant parts of your body.

Let's return to my moment of discovery during the surgical procedure in which I was involved as first assistant. The dime-sized *calcium plaque* had adhered to the outer surface of the *dura mater* at the back of the patient's neck about midway between the upper and lower ends. At the time of this surgery the patient was unable to walk or put pressure on the bottoms of his feet. We felt that this plaque would paralyze his legs if allowed to continue to grow. The surgical procedure was done with the patient secured on a special table. He lay on his stomach with his head tilted forward so that we could gain good access to the back of his neck. Our surgical incision ran on the midline at the back of his neck from just below the base of his skull to the lower neck. We separated muscles, retracting them to the left and to the right. When we reached the *vertebrae* (bones) of his *cervical* (neck) spine we removed enough of this bone to see the outer surface of the *dura mater (dural membrane)* and the dime-sized *calcium plaque* attached to it. The task now became to remove the plaque without damaging or cutting the membrane. To make a cut in the *dural membrane* would be to open an avenue for infection which could result in *spinal meningitis* or *encephalitis,* at worst. The *dura mater membrane* is a wonderful protective barrier for the brain and *spinal cord.* A cut in the *dural membrane* could also result in a leakage of *cerebrospinal fluid* from the inside of the membrane to the outside. If that condition persisted after surgery, a chronic deficiency of *cerebrospinal fluid* could occur.

At this point in the surgery my job was to hold the *dural membrane* very still with forceps placed about a quarter of an inch on each side of the *plaque.* With the membrane being held still, Jim the neurosurgeon would have an excellent chance of using his scalpel to remove the *calcium plaque* without cutting through the *dural membrane.*

To my consternation, frustration and embarrassment, this simple task of holding the *dural membrane* still proved to be impossible. It kept beating rhythmically, protruding from the operative site toward us and then withdrawing away from us. This activity of the *dural membrane* seemed to be cycling at a steady rate of between eight to ten cycles per minute. (I timed it with the operating room clock for several minutes.)

Further, I could clearly see the machine monitoring the patient's breathing, and I observed that the rhythmical activity of the *dural membrane* was not in synchrony with the patient's breathing. Nor was it in synchrony with the heart monitor, which was also within my view. As I continued unsuccessfully to try to hold this membrane still, ideas began to pop into my head about possible causes of its activity. The one idea that kept returning was that the membrane was responding to the rise and fall of fluid pressures on its inner side. This fluid would have to be *cerebrospinal fluid,* and, if this was true, the *cerebrospinal-fluid* pressure was rhythmically rising and falling at a rate of eight to ten cycles per minute. The amateur physicist in me immediately suggested that I was viewing a hydraulic system that was not described in any textbook I had ever read. I tried my idea out on Jim, but he had nothing to offer; neither did the anesthesiologist, the intern, nor any of the nurses. We completed the surgery. Jim was able to remove the plaque from the constantly moving membrane without mishap. He was a bit put out with me for being unable to successfully fulfill my role as the membrane stabilizer. On the other hand, he too was somewhat curious about the mechanism behind the *dural membrane's* motion. After the surgery, we talked about it some more, and Jim confessed that he had never noticed anything like this moving membrane in all his years of practice.

During the months that followed, the patient recovered full use of his feet. I continued to puzzle over the persistent rhythmical movement of the *dural membrane*. About six months later, I came across an advertisement in a professional journal that described a five-day hands-on seminar that was to be presented by a group of osteopathic physicians called The Cranial Academy. The advertisement alluded to the medically unconventional belief held in Cranial Osteopathy that the bones of the skull *move*. I wondered if this was related to the movement of the *dural membrane* we had observed. I discussed this possible relationship with Jim, and we decided I should attend the seminar.

The seminar's main topic turned out to be that skull bones exhibit a rhythmic movement as though they are responding to a hydraulic system, just as I had imagined during the surgery. I shared my experience and my similar view at the seminar. Some presenters had other theories that were much more fanciful than my idea of the hydraulic system, and the officials at the seminar were not receptive to the hydraulic system concept as I explained it. They did, however, have some good practical ideas about what could be done therapeutically by moving the skull bones. I combined their ideas with my own and brought them back to Jim.

In our discussions we decided that if I was right in thinking what we had observed involved a hydraulic system, then the container had to be waterproof with a little bit of stretchability, but not too much. It had to be strong and flexible. Since we had seen it in action, the container pretty much had to be the *dural membrane*. This membrane as a whole forms a watertight container shaped rather like a pollywog with its head in the skull and its tail running inside the canal within the spinal column. Inside the pollywog head is your brain. Traveling down inside the pollywog's tail is your *spinal cord*. The attachments of the *dural membrane* compartment make it watertight except in special areas where *cerebrospinal fluid* can flow in and out in a controlled way. In terms of physics, this qualifies the hydraulic system as "semi-closed"; that is, the fluid flows and rates of flow into and out of our pollywog-shaped *dural membrane* compartment are controlled. The control has to be by some body system. (At the time, this system was yet to be discovered.) The fluid that the container holds is *cerebrospinal fluid*.

Trying to Piece It Together

I puzzled a bit about why this semi-closed hydraulic system had not been seen before. Jim was quick to point out that in most cases of surgery involving the brain or spinal cord, the *dural membrane* is cut as a part of the surgical procedure. As soon as the *dural membrane* is cut, the rhythmical rise and fall of fluid pressure and volume is interrupted. The hydraulic system, in effect, has sprung a leak. Also, when we do *spinal taps,* we watch the *cerebrospinal-fluid* pressure go up the manometer (pressure measuring device) until it peaks. As soon as we reach that pressure peak we begin to drain some *cerebrospinal fluid* into test tubes to go to the laboratory for testing. After it peaks the pressure begins to decline. Usually we attribute this pressure drop to the removal of the *cerebrospinal-fluid* sample. This may be partially true, but the drop may also be at least partially due to the rhythmical rise and fall of *cerebrospinal-fluid* pressure within the *dural membrane* container.

Finally Some Support

After these events, I published a number of articles about our findings, but for some time I failed to receive any confirmation of them from other researchers. Finally I was deeply relieved by some correspondence I received from a professor of neurosurgery in Zurich, Switzerland. He had read some of my more technical writings regarding the *craniosacral system* and wished to support my observations with his own. He had done about twenty thousand surgeries on the brain and *spinal cord*— about eleven thousand on the brain and nine thousand on the *spinal cord.* He had observed the same rhythmical activity that I described involving the *dural membrane* before it is cut. He simply had never been curious about it since his surgical procedure generally demanded all of his concentration. This preoccupation with the surgery may explain why so many neurosurgeons who have had the opportunity to see the *craniosacral system* in action have failed to take note of it.

My First Patients

I came back from The Cranial Academy seminar with the concept that skull bones move in relationship to each other under normal circumstances throughout life. This was a departure from the concept taught in our medical schools that the bones of the skull start out as separate units when we are born, but soon fuse together so that by the time we reach puberty the skull is pretty much one solid bone, rather like a coconut.

I had felt the motion of skull bones with my own hands on several adult heads (my classmates) during the seminar and had no doubt that the classical ideas about skull bones fusing together early in life was incorrect. I coupled this newly attained manual skill (feeling skull bones moving in relationship to one another) with what I had seen at the surgical procedure with Jim. I then came up with my own ideas about how this new knowledge and manual skill might be applied to patients.

Jim supplied me with my first patient. He was the seven-year-old son of his office nurse. The boy had suffered for several years with pain in his ears. This pain was sometimes, but not always, accompanied by infection. The pain was caused by a buildup of fluid behind his eardrum in the middle-ear compartment. The ear specialist had inserted drainage tubes through his eardrums on three previous occasions. The tubes stayed in for a while but eventually either worked their way out or clogged up and became infected.

The boy was scheduled for another surgical insertion of these tubes into both eardrums just as I returned from The Cranial Academy seminar. Jim was concerned because each time a tube is inserted in the eardrum some of that eardrum's ability to respond to sound vibrations may be lost—the eardrum may get a little stiffer each time. Jim asked me if I had learned anything at the seminar that might help the boy avoid another surgery. I felt it was at least worth the effort to see if I could help, so I examined the boy's head by placing my hands gently in various positions to see if I could sense a problem with the movement of any of the skull bones. As I was examining, I understood clearly that the skull bones were moving rhythmically in response to the rise and fall of *cerebrospinalfluid* pressure within the boy's skull. It dawned on me that the skull-bone motion was a response to the rise and fall of *cerebrospinal-fluid* pressure and volume within its semi-closed hydraulic compartment, which was formed by the watertight outer layer of the *meningeal membranes,* the *dura mater.* So I visualized a hydraulic system inside the skull causing these bones to move rhythmically. If for some reason the skull bones were stuck and unable to accommodate the movement being "requested" by the hydraulic system, symptoms of some kind could be the result. In examining the boy's skull for rhythmical bone motion, I found that neither of his *temporal bones* was moving.

The *temporal bones* are paired one on each side of the head. They form the ear mountings and extend upwards perhaps two inches above the ear canal. They also have a horizontal component that extends inward and forms a part of the floor of the skull compartment.

The ear canals, *tympanic membranes* (eardrums), the middle- and inner-ear compartments, the hearing mechanisms, and the structures involved in our sense of equilibrium all reside within the *temporal bones.* The *eustachian tube* runs from the middle-ear compartment and drains into the back of the throat on each side. If these tubes do not function properly, the result is a buildup of fluid pressure behind the eardrum that causes a lot of pain and, in extreme cases, the need for the insertion of tubes through the eardrums to relieve the pressure.

Fluid in the middle-ear compartments is secreted by the linings of the compartments. It serves to cleanse these compartments. The fluid is supposed to drain through the *eustachian tubes* into the throat, keeping the tubes clean and clear as it passes through. These tubes pass through the lower parts of the *temporal bones* en route to their exits into the throat.

Perhaps the inability of the boy's *temporal bones* to move in response to the internal hydraulic system was related to the inability of the tubes to drain the middle-ear compartments. I sensed the *temporal bones'* inability to move, and I could feel the locations of the restrictions that were preventing bone motion. I put gentle force against the restrictions in synchrony with each expansion phase of the hydraulic system. My urging coupled with the fluid force from inside, which I patiently and gently continued through perhaps a hundred rhythmical cycles, ultimately liberated the *temporal bones,* and they began to move rhythmically in synchrony with the internal hydraulic system. Within a few hours the boy's mother called me and said that her son's pain was gone. The next day he was examined by the ear specialist. His *eustachian tubes* were now functional. The ear surgery was canceled. I remained in contact with the boy and his mother for about three years after this single treatment. There were no recurrences of the ear problems.

A second patient followed closely on the heels of that first one. This patient also came to me from Jim. The patient was a World War II veteran in his late fifties. He had been on disability since the war due to ringing in the ears and severe headaches, both of which were constant. He had been on tranquilizers and strong pain medication since the war. He had been in the Navy stationed aboard a battleship. The noise of an explosion gave him a sudden pain in his head, which was accompanied very shortly after by a ringing in his ears. He had lived with this problem for about thirty years. He had found no relief since the explosion, except by the use of his medications, which took the edge off the pain and softened the ringing in his ears. But as the medications wore off, the pain and ringing increased. Even with heavy doses of medication he was never completely symptom-free. He found Jim in his search for help, and Jim asked me to try out this new "stuff" on this poor suffering veteran.

I did the same thing I did with the boy. In this case it felt like both of his *temporal bones* were pushed in towards the center of his head and were "stuck" there. They were not moving at all. In addition, I found the base of his skull where it meets his neck was very tight, and the skull bone back there, the *occiput,* was pulled forward. It also felt like his forehead and the *occiput* were being pulled towards each other by an elastic connection. So in essence, this man's whole skull felt to me as though it was being contracted inward, both side-to-side and front-to-back. However, the bones on the top of his head, the *parietal bones,* were moving in an attempt to accommodate the internal fluctuations in *cerebrospinal-fluid* rhythmical pressure.

I started by trying to exaggerate the rhythmical motion of the *parietal bones;* gradually, I was able to establish some front-to-back mobility. As that increased, I broadened my focus to releasing the side-to-side inward contraction. It took about ten hours of hands-on work over a five-day period to mobilize this man's skull to a point of reasonable restoration. To my amazement his symptoms improved during the ten hours of treatment, and by the end he was symptom-free and drug-free. The patient, Jim the neurosurgeon, and I were all astounded. This seemed impossible, but here it was before our very eyes.

A Therapy Is Born

These two experiences with patients very much hooked me on what I saw as a developing treatment process. It was an amalgamation of my surgical experience and what I'd learned at The Cranial Academy seminar. Jim was also hooked, and he suggested that I begin to work with his brain-surgery patients on the first day after surgery. It was quite a scary idea for me, but nonetheless a tempting one. Jim was very reassuring.

Together we reasoned that boosting the performance of the internal, semi-closed hydraulic *cerebrospinal-fluid* system could enhance brain-surgery recovery. We felt it was important to act as soon after surgery as possible.

Jim selected patients he thought would not be risky for me to work on. I also began serving as Jim's first assistant during surgery so that I would become familiar with what was done. That would help me create the most effective approach to hands-on treatment. I began treating two or three of Jim's brain-surgery patients per week. Jim kept score, and after a few weeks he informed me that recovery was much quicker, complications were fewer, and post-surgical disabilities were reduced. We were both walking on air.

Time passed and both Jim and I began to gain a reputation for doing this "weird stuff" that didn't have a name yet. It was very different in conception and application from what I learned from The Cranial Academy, but it did incorporate some of the Academy's ideas; namely, that the skull bones move. Besides, it was at The Cranial Academy seminar where I found that I could and should trust what my hands told me, even if it con-flicted with the American and British anatomy books. And my hands told me that the skull bones do indeed move. I found out later that Italian anatomy books teach that skull bones do not fuse under normal circumstances. Medical teachings, it turns out, aren't written in stone—there is another way of looking at things. What my hands are able to feel has become a great source of understanding about many things, not the least of which is this semi-closed hydraulic system that we soon would dub the *"craniosacral system."*

Proof: The Skull Bones Do Not Fuse

In July 1975 I accepted a faculty position as a clinician researcher at Michigan State University's Department of Biomechanics. I remained there doing research for about eight-and-one-half years. During that time we proved that skull bones do not fuse. Here's how that came about.

The joints between skull bones are called *"sutures."* These *sutures* are full of elastic fibers, nonelastic *collagen* fibers, lots of blood vessels, and nerve endings. The misinformation about bones fusing together had its basis in the study of anatomy laboratory cadavers that were old and embalmed. The changes in the *suture* that look like fusing or calcification occur after death, not before. We discovered this by studying bone and *suture* samples taken from living adults of all ages during brain surgery.

Another thing we discovered was that we can *stop* the movement of the skull bones by pressing on the tailbone very gently. We learned this by working with live monkeys. We observed that the hydraulic system is in fact continuous from head to tail. That prompted us to name it the *"craniosacral system."* This work was done with neurophysiologist Ernest Retzlaff, PhD. The next logical step was to name the treatment process. We chose "CranioSacral Therapy."

Working with a biophysicist, Zvi Karni, PhD, DSc, we then discovered that when CranioSacral Therapy releases restrictions of the *craniosacral system*, there is a significant change in the electrical potential of the whole body. The activity of the electrical baseline smooths out and drops to a lower potential. We also discovered that, along with the change in electrical potential, there is a temporary stopping of the *craniosacral system's* rhythmical activity.

We called this stopping a "Significance Detector" because, when this sort of stoppage occurs, it is a sign that the patient's body is doing something positive and significant. It also signals to the therapist that he or she is on the right track. It was wonderful to get confirmation from electrical measuring devices that what my hands were telling me was true. Later we found that it was possible and beneficial to induce this stoppage as a part of CranioSacral Therapy. In this case we call the stoppage a "*still point*," and the process by which the stoppage is intentionally produced "Still-Point Induction."

Autism

We did a lot of basic scientific work on the *craniosacral system* and then branched into research with children suffering from brain dysfunction. I spent three years at a Center for Autism researching that problem with Jon Vredevoogd, a design specialist, and several graduate students. We found that we could differentiate *autistic* children from *schizophrenic* children by the evaluation of their *craniosacral system* functions.

Both *autistic* and *schizophrenic* children had minimal movement of the bones of the skull upon evaluation. The lack of skull-bone movement in the autistic children appeared to be due to a particular inability of the membranes of the *craniosacral system* to expand with the fluid-filling phase of the system. The outer layer of the *dural membrane* in the skull is the attached lining of the inner side of the skull bones. When the membrane is too tight, the bones are held snugly in a contracted position and the *sutures* (the joints between the skull bones) cannot expand.

We found that we could not expand these *suture* joints by

trying to slide the two contributing bones away from each other. It was fairly easy to see that *autistic* children, for some reason, have *dural membranes* that lack the elasticity needed to accommodate fluctuations in fluid volume and pressure in their *craniosacral systems.*

In contrast, despite minimal skull-bone motion in *schizophrenic* children, our gentle manual urgings were able to induce movement. The *suture* joints were not physically or structurally restricted. Instead, it seemed there was not enough inherent energy within the *craniosacral system* to create the rhythmical skull-bone motion to which we had become accustomed. Could *schizophrenia* be a disorder in which there is something inherently wrong in the *craniosacral system?* That's a conclusion I reached early on; though sadly, it seems that CranioSacral Therapy can do little to correct it. With *autism,* however, it turns out there is much we can do.

From the CranioSacral Therapist's perspective it seemed that if we stretched the *autistic* child's membranes, there would be plenty of energy in the *craniosacral system* to set up the rhythmical activity we were hoping for. So we set out to work with *autistic* children. This was a very challenging task. Most *autistic* children do not like to be touched. Many like to press very hard on the roofs of their mouths with their thumbs. This pressure interferes with the workings of the *craniosacral system,* so the thumbs couldn't be in their mouths while we did our work. Other *autistic* children like to chew very hard on their wrists or at the base of the thumbs. That had to stop too. It took weeks of work to get cooperation from each child. We did it by blending in with their world and letting them feel very gentle hand placement wherever they would allow it. We had to make friends and *earn* each child's trust. It took several months of once-a-week appointments to begin to apply Cranio-

Sacral Therapy effectively. When this finally occurred, we found that when we were able to stretch the membranes in front of the skull away from the back, the child voluntarily stopped pressing on the roof of his/her mouth and quit chewing on the wrist or thumb. This led me to consider that these so-called *"autistic"* activities were just the child's attempt to loosen tightness inside the skull by head banging and pressing on the roof of the mouth. Now, when your head is compressed it hurts. I suspected that the wrist and thumb chewing were the child's attempt to create pain that he/she was in control of in order to overshadow the head pain over which there was no control. Also, the chewing may have stimulated the production of natural body *analgesics (endorphins),* which would then bring relief from all pains.

As we continued our work with *autistic* children, we noted that decompressing the head, one side away from the other, resulted in behavioral changes that were very favorable. These children who were known for their avoidance of human inter-relationships, who preferred to have a love affair with an inanimate object, suddenly began to hug us, to kiss us, and to come to us. This was essentially unknown for *autistic* children.

As we were able to further decompress, they began to express various emotions related to anger and/or fear. Once this was over, some of them seemed to be quite normal for a time, but then regressed back into *autism.* I believe this regression occurred as the growth of the brain and skull bones used up the "slack" we had created in the *dural membranes.* The brain once again came under pressure and the *autistic* symptoms returned. These children would need ongoing treatment to continue stretching the *dural membranes* in order to stay ahead of the brain and bone growth that was genetically controlled. We did have a few ongoing success stories, but the follow-up care for most of the children we treated was not available after our research contract expired.

When It Works, It Works

One of our success stories was a five-year-old boy who was diagnosed as *autistic* by the Navy doctors in Norfolk, Virginia. The father was a Navy man at the time. The diagnosis of *autism* was confirmed at the University of Virginia. Following this the father received a hardship discharge from the Navy. The family returned to their home state, Michigan, in order to begin a new life centered around the best possible care for their *autistic* son. The Michigan evaluation team from the state educational system confirmed the diagnosis of *autism*. The boy was brought to me at the University clinic as a private patient. He was not a participant in our official research program at the Center for Autism. I treated this boy five times, releasing the front-to-back and side-to-side restrictions quite easily. His *autism* had only appeared about a year earlier. His response to the CranioSacral approach was excellent. His *dural membranes* released and he was apparently quite normal by the third treatment. Treatment sessions four and five revealed no return of the membranous restrictions, nor of the skull-bone immobilizations that typically appeared secondary to the membranous restrictions of the *dura mater*. The boy was re-evaluated by the Michigan evaluation team. He was deemed normal. The previous diagnoses by the Naval doctors, the University of Virginia pediatric psychiatrist, and the same Michigan evaluation team were considered erroneous. No one wanted to believe that a case of *autism* could be cured in just a few weeks with about five hours of hands-on CranioSacral Therapy. This boy remained quite normal for the three years that his parents and I maintained contact. I believe the problem was permanently solved.

A Touching Case

Another boy, age sixteen, who was at the Center for Autism, completely normalized as he was treated on a weekly basis as a participant in our research project. This boy was totally withdrawn and mute when we began our work with him. He was very well-developed and about six feet tall. Initially, he would come into the treatment room and get into a fetal position under the treatment table. Our treatment table was a simple nonportable massage table. For this project our treatment sessions were about thirty minutes in duration. He would come in and curl up under the table and remain there during the entire thirty minutes. We (my graduate students, of which there were usually three or four present, and myself) would then very carefully and tenderly place our hands on his body wherever he would allow it. I usually focused upon trying to halt the *craniosacral rhythm* activity (a Still-Point Induction) by my touch. I will explain how you can perform this technique as an amateur later in this book.

We continued to work with him in this way. I recall quite specifically that during his fourth session he voluntarily came out from under the treatment table and lay down on top of the table. I placed my hands on his head. He placed his hands upon mine and moved them to a slightly different position with which he seemed quite happy. I had four graduate students with me that day. I instructed them each to gently place their hands on one of the boy's limbs and to gently lift it a few inches above the tabletop. My purpose was to allow the patient's arms and legs to be free of gravity and tabletop friction.

Soon the legs and arms were tending to move into various motion patterns. I instructed the graduate students to follow these movements as sensitively as they could. Soon the session was over, and our sixteen-year-old *autistic* boy got up from the table and, without a word or a side look, walked very quickly to the door and left the room.

The next week he came into the room, quickly walked to the treatment table and lay down. I made my hands available to him. He took my hands and placed them precisely where he wanted them, one on each side of his head with the heels of my palms about an inch apart and with the front-to-back midline dividing the space between them. I noted that my hands were very symmetrically placed upon his head. The same four graduate students were with me during this session, and we picked up almost precisely where we had left off the previous week. This time the patient guided me to twist the two sides of his head in opposite directions as you might wring out a wet washcloth. As we did this, I realized we were working at the release of his temporal bones and the related side-to-side compression of his skull. As this progressed, the arms and legs went into a wide variety of rather bizarre positions and contortions that were supported against gravity and expertly followed by each of the graduate students, one on each limb.

This went on for about twenty minutes. Then he returned to a rather neutral position, lying on his back on the table. His guidance of my hands relaxed, and I simply followed his *craniosacral system's* activity in his head as gently and unintrusively as I could. In a moment or two he sat up as if to leave the treatment room. I asked him to please sit a moment while we videotaped his facial expression. He looked totally at peace. I wanted this expression on tape. As I put my hands on his shoulders, he very gently put his right hand on my face. He pulled me into position so that our faces were side-by-side, then he turned and kissed me gently and lovingly on my left cheek. Then he left the treatment area.

A week later he came in smiling, lay down on the table, accepted treatment, and gave me yes and no head movements in response to my questions. I asked him if he could speak. He had not uttered a word thus far in our relationship. He shook his head no in answer to my question. I asked if there was something wrong with his physical ability to form words; he nodded yes. I asked him to point to the place where the trouble was, if he knew. He pointed to his Adam's apple.

We became good friends. He learned to sign and attempted to teach us a few simple sign-language words. I recommended that he be evaluated by a throat specialist. We saw him three more times before he was removed from the Center for Autism because he was no longer *autistic*. He was called a "spontaneous remission" by the director of the center.

It seems that *autistic* children may outgrow the condition, either by turning into *"schizophrenics"* or by "normalizing." It was a joy to work with this boy. I have difficulty accepting the idea that he would have "normalized" whether or not he had seen us. I never heard what happened with his speech deficit, but I do hope that the specialists were able to help him. He was, and I presume is, a kind and loving human being.

Further Explorations

In addition to our work at the Center for Autism, I opened a clinic for brain-dysfunctioning children on campus at Michigan State University. Here we received patients suffering from a very wide array of problems, including *paralyses* of all types due to a variety of causes ranging from birth trauma to *cerebral palsy, spinal cord* injuries, head injuries, *nerve root compressions,* and so on. We also saw a large number of *seizure* problems—*grand mal, petit mal, temporal lobe, single-limb convulsions,* and so on. There were *hyperkinetic disorders, attention deficit disorders, dyslexia, dyscalculia,* and a wide variety of retardation problems. There were also a lot of speech and motor-deficit problems.

Our research had shown strong correlations between specific problems of the *craniosacral system's* function and the child's performance in school. Many of the children with the most significant *craniosacral system* dysfunctions had suffered obstetrically complicated deliveries, such as prolonged labor, often coupled with breech, face, arm, shoulder or footling presentations; pharmaceutical induction of labor; forceps deliveries of all kinds; and *Caesarean section* deliveries. It was easy to understand the stress induced in most of these delivery problems, with the exception of *Caesarean section.*

Our research with grade-school children showed that C-section babies seemed to have a large number of *craniosacral system* problems. An idea presented itself to me during a conversation with a pathologist who was describing his observations on stillborn babies. He said that many stillborn babies showed abnormal strain patterns in the *meningeal membrane system* inside the skull. These strain patterns were indicated by the presence of small areas of bleeding, as though the membranes had been stressed and stretched to the point of rupturing some of the small blood vessels, particularly within the *dural membrane.*

At this point in our conversation it dawned on me that when we do *Caesarean sections* we often make a *sudden* cut into the pregnant *uterus* because we are in a hurry to deliver an infant in distress. When we make that quick cut, the fluid inside the *uterus* often squirts two or three inches into the air. This squirting of *amniotic fluid* out of the *uterus* through the incision indicates that there is a rapid lowering of fluid pressure inside the *uterus.* The baby is subjected to this sharp pressure reduction. This situation would cause the infant's head to expand rapidly. At that stage of development the bones of the skull have not yet formed the *sutures*. The various bones are connected via *dural membranes*. Sudden expansion of the skull might very well cause strain of the *dural membrane* system within the skull.

Along with the strain in this kind of tissue there is often a tearing of some of the tiny blood vessels within the membrane. When this occurs, red blood cells leak out into the membrane tissue. These blood cells deteriorate because they are in a non-supporting environment outside the blood vessels. Their deterioration produces irritating, slightly toxic substances, which cause the membranes to become less compliant and supple. These membranes respond to the irritants by becoming more *fibrous,* similar to the scars when your skin is cut or torn, but not quite as severe. These areas of increased *fibrous* tissue that develop within the *dural membranes* can be the cause of problems with the function of the *craniosacral system* as that system develops and grows. This seems a reasonable explanation for the high correlation we found in grade-school children between multiple *craniosacral system* problems and history of *Caesarean section* deliveries.

As our on-campus clinic for brain-dysfunctioning children developed, we saw general improvement in almost all the children we treated. Children receiving CranioSacral Therapy for specific problems also became less susceptible to infections such as colds, *bronchitis,* and the like. They also became more tolerant of things to which they had previously been considered allergic. This was especially true in the areas of intolerance for various foods and sugar. Sleeping habits improved, and children troubled by constipation improved significantly.

Parents reported all these changes as they came in with their children, usually on a weekly, bi-weekly or, less often, monthly basis. Other reports from parents were almost universally related to improvements in general attitude, morale, mental alertness and sense of humor. These were all changes in general well-being that were not necessarily the considerations that brought the children to the CranioSacral Therapy clinic initially.

In treating patients with *paralysis*, we found that in spastic cases due to *cerebral palsy*, we were quite successful in reducing or eliminating the *spasticity*. The muscle-relaxing change almost always increased the child's level of comfort. It is uncomfortable and often quite painful when muscles are chronically spastic. These muscles may also be "hair-triggered" so that they over-respond to small stimuli by "cramping." We had some experiences wherein the reduction of *spasticity* was enough to reverse the *paralysis*.

Some of these children began to use paralyzed limbs for walking, picking up objects, etc. In other cases the reduction of *spasticity* did not help the *paralysis*. The previously spastic limb or body part was now soft and pliable, but still not under voluntary control of the child. In any case, the reduction did represent a significant improvement, if only in comfort. In *paralysis* of the lower body due to spinal injuries, we had a significant number of successes.

In order to get this kind of positive result, it was essential that the *spinal cord* still be intact, that it had not been severed by the trauma. Other cases of paralysis involved such things as *Erb's palsy*, a condition in which the nerves to the arm are compressed, usually due to some birthing injury, and the arm and hand are essentially useless to the child. Our success with these children was quite good in terms of the restoration of function.

In all cases we saw that the sooner we got to the child after the onset of the *paralysis,* the better the chances would be of a good result. I still find it difficult to predict which *paralysis* cases will respond favorably to CranioSacral Therapy; however, since our treatment is essentially risk-free and we can count on a significant improvement in general health, morale, and sense of well-being, I can see no reason not to give Cranio-Sacral Therapy a try, no matter what the cause or the age.

An Exhilarating Case

As an example of attempting treatment on a trial basis, I am, as of this writing (1999), still working with a sixty-eight-year-old man who was born with *Erb's palsy* that resulted in the lack of development of his left arm and hand. He came to us in about 1993 because of constant pain in his left shoulder, upper back and neck. His left arm and hand were infantile in development. His left arm muscles, involving the elbow and upper arm, were very tight and did not allow him to straighten his arm more than about sixty degrees at the elbow. He had undergone two surgeries on the left shoulder to eliminate the pain. They were successful in releasing his left upper arm and shoulder enough so that his arm was not as twisted or drawn across his chest as it had been, but the pain was still there.

We were able to relieve the pain using a combination of CranioSacral Therapy and some spinal mobilization techniques. After a few months he noticed he was getting some movement in the fingers of his left hand. This seemed quite unlikely since the hand had neither developed nor moved voluntarily since his birth. His family doctor confirmed the progress, however. He also reported that it appeared as though the skin of the arm and hand was looking more vital. All of us had our curiosity piqued.

The patient lives about a thousand miles from our Institute in Palm Beach Gardens, Florida, but he comes to us for treatment about two or three days every few months. Since we began going beyond the treatment of pain, we have seen his arm grow and his left hand become partially functional. We also have X-ray documentation of bone growth and healthy development. These are things that were genetically scheduled to occur years ago. We have released the *dural membrane* tensions, mobilized his spine, and induced, by the use of our hands only, the transmission of nerve influences from the brain-control areas into his left arm and hand.

These results are astonishing even to me. This man's body seems to remember what it wanted to do more than sixty years ago, but could not. The plan is still in place, and he is rapidly developing the arm that he was meant to have at birth. What does it hurt to try? You never know what these wonderful bodies of ours might be able to accomplish given a little help and encouragement by a skillful CranioSacral Therapist.

Seizures and Hyperkinesis

Seizures were another problem that we saw a lot of in our CranioSacral Therapy clinic at Michigan State University. Our success with *seizures* was quite respectable, and it followed a bell-curve distribution. There were a few *seizure* children who received no help at all from CranioSacral Therapy, but no harm was done either. There were also a few children who, within the range of ten to twenty treatments, were able to become *seizure*-free. In my opinion, it is a real boon to reduce *seizure*-suppressant medication whenever possible, especially in children. Childhood is a time when so much learning is going on and so many brain circuits are being developed that it seems a shame to suppress brain activity, even a little bit, by the use of medication. We will never know what the child might have been had he or she not required *seizure*-suppressant medication; even so, it seems prudent to me to reduce medication levels whenever and wherever possible.

I believe that a significant number of *seizure* problems are the result of abnormal *dural membrane* tension within the skull. These abnormal tensions can interfere with the normal delivery of both blood and *cerebrospinal fluid* to given brain areas. The dural tensions can also place pressure and/or strain upon brain tissue, *per se*. Brain tissue relies upon the conduction of very tiny and delicate electrical currents along nerve fibers that depend upon a very precisely balanced and controlled environment in order to do their job. When pressure is placed on the brain tissue by the membrane, or blood circulation is impaired, or *cerebrospinal-fluid* supply is not adequate, the nerves cannot do their job properly. If the nerve cell bodies are accumulating electrical energy that the fibers cannot easily conduct, the energy builds up in the nerve cells. Ultimately, the buildup of energy goes so high that it explodes in an uncontrolled way and travels on whichever fibers will carry it out into the fluid that surrounds it. This fluid also has electrical conductor qualities, so the fluid spreads the exploding electrical energy to adjacent nerve cells that may not be affected by the pressure or compromised blood and *cerebrospinal-fluid* supply. These adjacent nerve cells may be stimulated to send off their impulses by the "electrified" field, and so it goes. The result is like a dam that is holding back the accumulated electrical energy from breaking. The result is *seizure*. If the *seizure* problem of the child is wholly or in part due to any of the factors described, CranioSacral Therapy can help. I think that quite often the causal factors I have mentioned are secondary contributors. That is why in the majority of *seizure* patients we get significant partial improvement with CranioSacral Therapy. When it completely eradicates the cause, it seems miraculous. Let me illustrate.

The mother of a four-year-old child called me from a hospital in the Midwest. The call came on a Thursday afternoon. The mother was absolutely frantic. Her son was scheduled for brain surgery on the following Tuesday. The child was suffering from almost constant *seizure* activity that had not responded to any medications. Many had been tried. The surgical plan was to cut the connections of the *left temporal lobe* of the brain, where the *seizures* originated, to the rest of the brain; this would isolate the *seizure* source so that the child would not continue to have "whole brain" *seizures*. The possibility was also mentioned to the mother that they might have to remove the *left temporal lobe*. This was what the mother heard, but she may have misinterpreted in her distraught and panicky condition. In any case, the situation was quite serious. They flew to our Institute on Thursday night. I saw the boy on Friday morning. The membranes were extremely strained in the region of the *left temporal lobe*. I was able to obtain a release of these membranes on Friday. We did more work on Monday and Tuesday. On Wednesday, he went home with his parents in a *seizure*-free state on a small dose of medication. Today he receives follow-up CranioSacral Therapy from a practitioner in their vicinity. His body continues to require some medication, but surgery is no longer a consideration. I am guessing that as time passes, the need for medication will disappear.

As our university clinic flourished, the number of learning-disabled children coming to us grew tremendously. We saw larger numbers of children who were diagnosed as *hyperkinetic*. This was in the late 1970s when that term was in vogue.

Today these children would be called ADD *(attention deficit disorder)* or ADHD *(attention deficit hyperactive disorder)*. We found that when the back of the skull was compressed against the top of the neck in a *hyperkinetic* child and we corrected this problem, the *hyperkinesis* would disappear. We had children who had to be held on the treatment table by their parents while I worked on them. When I got the release at the base of the skull, more often than not the child fell asleep on the table. Usually this problem had to be corrected four or five times to make the improvement permanent, but it was really a pretty easy problem for CranioSacral Therapy to handle. It is also interesting that most of these children were on the Feingold diet at that time. After the CranioSacral correction, the dietary restrictions were no longer necessary. I would estimate that about two-thirds of the children with the diagnosis of *hyperkinesis* presented the problem of compression of the back of the skull onto the upper neck. I would venture to say that all of the children with this problem responded favorably when the correction was accomplished. The other one-third of the *hyperkinetic* children had other causes for their behavior that did not fall within the realm of the CranioSacral Therapy practitioner. This observation led me to suggest to the university psychology department that hyperkinesis could be subdivided into cases being due to *craniosacral system* dysfunction, emotional causes, allergic causes, and so on. My point was that a simple examination by a CranioSacral Therapy practitioner could sort out the children who would most likely respond to our treatment and those who would not. I felt these subcategories would be helpful, but no one in authority took note.

Hyperactivity Explained

My concept of *hyperkinetic* behavior is really quite simple. I see it as related to the compression of the base of the skull *(occipital bone)* into the top of the neck, as I mentioned in the last section. The *occipital bone* and the paired *temporal bones,* located just forward of the *occiput,* meet to form a part of the floor of the skull just behind and below the ear canals. Moving in towards the center of the skull about an inch on each side, there are gaps between these two bones. These gaps, one on each side, are round-oval in shape and about one-quarter-inch in diameter in a grade-school child. These gaps are called the *"jugular foramina."* Through these *foramina* pass the *jugular veins,* one on each side, and three major *cranial nerves.* The nerves are *glossopharyngeal,* the *vagus* and *spinal accessory.* The *jugular veins* drain seventy-five to eighty-five percent of the blood from the head.

What we have found in our craniosacral *hyperkinetic* children is that the *occiput* is jammed forward upon the top *cervical vertebra* (the *atlas*) and is maintained in this abnormal position by contracture of muscles that connect the back of the head to the neck. These layers of muscle run vertically and are about an inch to an inch-and-a-half thick in preadolescent children. When they contract to maintain the malposition of the *occiput* on the *atlas,* I believe it is a protective device aimed at prevention of further forward slippage of the occiput. If the occiput slips to the point of impinging upon the *spinal cord,* it is devastating and life-threatening.

I would speculate that most of these forward malpositions of the *occiput* are due to birth trauma as the head is pulled face down under the mother's pubic bones by the obstetrical delivery person in an effort to speed the delivery process. Some-

times the *occiput* moves back where it belongs. Sometimes a
bit of panic may set in, and the infant reflexively contracts
these muscles, which then stay that way. When this occurs, the
passage of the *jugular veins* through the *jugular foramina* may
be narrowed somewhat. This, in turn, compromises the flow
of blood through these *jugular veins* to some degree. It requires
a little extra "back" pressure to keep this drainage system
going.

This back pressure reflects into the child's head and does
two things. First, it increases the pressure inside his or her skull
to a small extent. But a little extra pressure on a brain can irri-
tate it a lot. When your brain is irritated it may be hard to con-
centrate and to sit still and obey the classroom rules. Second,
the back-pressure drainage may slightly reduce the inflow of
fresh blood to the brain. The new blood can't get in easily if
the old blood is having trouble vacating the premises. By "new"
blood I mean blood that is fresh and full of oxygen. Old blood
has delivered its oxygen and now carries carbon dioxide and
waste products. Both of these factors could contribute to an
irritable and *hyperkinetic* brain in a child with attention deficit
disorder.

As an aside, the same compression in newborns often causes
the *vagus nerve,* which passes through the *jugular foramina,*
to act abnormally. Since the *vagus nerve* is strongly influen-
tial in stomach, bowel, gallbladder and swallow functions, we
find that infants with colic and *esophageal reflux* respond
extremely well to CranioSacral Therapy when the muscles at
the base of the skull and the upper neck are abnormally tight.

Reading Problems (Dyslexia and Dyscalculia)

We also treated a large number of children with reading problems in our university clinic. Once again, the language has

changed since the late 1970s. At that time these children were diagnosed as *dyslexic*. At present the term *"dyslexia"* is in a state of transition, and I have seen that it means somewhat different things to different authorities. In any case, the children we treated had trouble reading. Most were reversing letter sequences, but there were exceptions. We found that when the *right temporal bone* was not moving freely, release of its restrictions would often result in improved reading skills. *Temporal bones* house the ear canal, inner ear and balance mechanisms.

Probably the most dramatic case I ever saw involved a fifteen-year-old boy who was about six feet tall and weighed in the vicinity of two hundred pounds. His teacher personally brought him to our clinic at the university. She told me that he was reading at a fourth-grade level. He was very frustrated and becoming very angry; he was rebellious towards authority and was beginning to threaten violence. I evaluated the boy and found his *right temporal bone* to be totally locked or stuck. I was able to mobilize it pretty well at our first treatment session. They made an appointment to return in two weeks.

When they returned I did not ask nor did they volunteer information about any changes in his condition, but his *right temporal bone* was almost normal. I completed that work and gave him a general mobilizing and balancing treatment aimed at the rehabilitation of his *craniosacral system,* which had apparently been trying to compensate for the immovable *right temporal bone* for some time. His body responded well to this treatment, but he said nothing to me, and I felt it better not to force conversation at the time.

In two weeks they returned for another appointment. I evaluated and further treated his *craniosacral system*. When I was finished, his teacher asked me how he was. I replied that the problem I had found initially in his *craniosacral system* was now fine, and that I did not believe there was any more I could do for him. The teacher now informed me that over the past four weeks since our first appointment, he had progressed from reading at a fourth-grade level to a tenth-grade level. She spoke about "miracles," about "never having seen anything like this before," and so on. I thanked her and assured her that I was not a miracle worker, that I was only using CranioSacral Therapy.

I then asked the boy what had changed for him. He replied that before the first treatment he could only "see" three or four letters at a time. If the word had more than four letters, he first had to memorize the letter sequence, then search his memory for the word. This kind of reading was very hard work. He hated it and was very angry that he had not been able to keep up with the other children his age since the time he was seven or eight years old.

Now he could see three or four words at a time, as well as long words of two or three syllables. He didn't have to memorize letter sequences. He was actually enjoying reading now. He felt good. He thanked me, his teacher thanked me, and they left. I got a Christmas card from him about eight months later. He thanked me again and said that he was doing very well.

This case was outstanding in terms of response. We had many more who improved significantly. I'm sure that for a child with any kind of reading difficulty, CranioSacral Therapy is worth a try. Done reasonably well there is no risk to the child.

We only had three cases of *dyscalculia*—the reversal of number sequences as they are perceived to be printed or written on paper. All three cases had *left temporal bone* restrictions. This was the opposite side from the *dyslexic* children, but the nature of the restriction was similar. It was simply a mirror image of what we saw in reading problems. Sadly, we were not able to see improvement in the arithmetic skills of any of the three *dyscalculic* children we treated, even though the *left temporal bone* restriction was corrected.

In all honesty, I have no theory I consider worthwhile to explain the good results in our CranioSacral Therapy treatment of reading problems by mobilizing the *right temporal bone*. Further, I have no theory as to why the three *dyscalculic* children presented essential mirror-image *temporal bone restrictions* on the left side. Nor do I understand why we were unable to help the *dyscalculic* children. I do know that CranioSacral Therapy helped about eighty percent of the more than fifty *dyslexic* children we treated in our clinic.

Developmental Delay

We also treated a large number of children with developmental delay problems, *mental retardation, microcephaly, hydrocephalus,* brain injury due to oxygen deprivation, *postencephalitis syndrome,* and just about anything you might imagine. In general, I have to say that each case is different. We evaluate the *craniosacral system* and treat what we find. Sometimes the results are dramatically positive, and very often we see some improvement in general comfort, sleep patterns and bowel function, as well as reduction in angry outbursts.

A Model Social Program

During the time I was working in the university clinic, one of the state directors of special education informed me that he estimated that five percent of all the children in the Michigan public school system were suffering some sort of brain func-

tion problem. The range of these dysfunctions included learning disabilities, *seizures,* developmental delay, *autism,* and
Down syndrome. At that time—around 1978—my research
was suggesting to me that all of these brain-dysfunctioning
children should receive *craniosacral system* evaluations, and
that about half of those would benefit from treatment. I actually believed that about two-and-one-half percent of *all* the
school children in the state of Michigan would do well to
receive some form of CranioSacral Therapy.

The size of this task, were it to be performed correctly, was
very scary, but I felt that it had to be done. After some deep
thought, I devised a training program to develop the therapists
we would need for this statewide work. Then I went to the
university curriculum committee. I was able to gain approval
for a graduate course in CranioSacral Therapy that covered
two academic quarters. The requirements for entry into the
course were set at having a license to do hands-on treatment
or to offer healthcare to other human beings. Thus, we wel-
comed practitioners of all kinds—dentists, nurses, physical
therapists, occupational therapists, massage therapists, aids to
all of the above, and, with special permission, psychologists
and special-education teachers.

During the first quarter we taught evaluation of the *craniosacral system*, and during the second we presented uncompli-
cated treatment techniques. It was a hands-on course wherein
the enrollees practiced techniques on each other under super-
vision after the theory had been discussed and the techniques
demonstrated. The class met for three hours at a time, two
evenings per week. Three graduate credits were given each
quarter to those who successfully completed the course. I was
very pleased at the progress that most of the enrollees made.
It demonstrated clearly that one did not need an advanced

medical education in order to do CranioSacral Therapy.

The work proved to be essentially risk-free, even in the hands of psychologists and special-education teachers without medical training. What is required to be a competent Cranio-Sacral Therapist is sensitivity, dedication, patience, and the ability to watch positive results occur even when you don't know how or why they are happening. This was the beginning of the use of a powerful but safe healthcare modality by nonphysicians.

Soon the graduates of the CranioSacral Therapy class began to work with children in the schools. Whenever they encountered *craniosacral system* problems that did not respond to simple treatment techniques, these caregivers would bring the children to our clinic for consultation and evaluation. There I had a chance not only to examine the patients, but also to see how the therapists were doing. I was again very favorably impressed. On the whole, our program seemed like a model that could be duplicated elsewhere in the state in order to get the treatment to the children who might benefit from the CranioSacral approach.

Once this program was underway, I began teaching Cranio-Sacral Therapy in England, France and Belgium. Its popularity grew very rapidly, and I spent about four to six weeks each summer for about six consecutive years teaching in Europe. Ultimately I helped to establish children's CranioSacral Therapy clinics in London and Brussels. In France they did not centralize a clinic, but many physical therapists and osteopaths offered CranioSacral Therapy in their private practices. The results reported by European practitioners of CranioSacral Therapy were quite excellent. And I personally enjoyed some successes with children while teaching in Europe.

No Miracles, Just CranioSacral Therapy

On one occasion I was conducting a CranioSacral Therapy seminar in Nice, France. One of the Belgian enrollees asked if I would treat a four-and-a-half-year-old boy whose mother had brought him from Brussels on the chance that I might see him. My policy was to decline private appointments because the rigors of teaching a hands-on class as the only instructor for about nine hours a day for five days did not leave much energy for after-hours private appointments. I did offer to demonstrate the classwork on the boy for each of the five days in front of the whole class. The mother accepted my offer. The boy was spastic and essentially paralyzed on his right side. Both his arm and his leg were involved. He wore very thick-lensed glasses and was severely cross-eyed. I was told that he could only swallow foods that had been pureed because he could not chew and swallow effectively; this had been the case since birth. His official diagnosis was *cerebral palsy*. The mother believed that he was okay at birth but had been injured in the hospital nursery. She believed this because the first day after delivery he had seemed fine to her. The next day, however, he was rather soft and flaccid and did not nurse effectively.

On the first day of the seminar I went through the introductory material and then used the boy to demonstrate the hands-on techniques to the class. I did the same thing with more advanced material on the second and third days of the seminar. On this third day I was demonstrating a release technique for the *suture* that runs across the top of the head about one-third of the way back from the forehead. This technique releases the *frontal bone* (which forms the forehead) from the *parietal bones* (which form the crown of the head). The *suture* between the *frontal bone* and the *parietal bones* is named the "*coronal suture.*" The boy's *coronal suture* was severely jammed. During the demonstration to the class I was able to effectively mobilize this jammed *suture*.

On the fourth day late in the afternoon, the students began cheering, standing on chairs, clapping, and in general not paying the least bit of attention to *me,* the professor! After a few seconds I saw what the cheering was about. The boy was here for his demonstration treatment. This time his mother was not carrying him. She was holding his hand! For the first time in his young life he was walking. Frankly, I was speechless. When I returned to Michigan, the mother brought her son to me for follow-up treatment. Within a month his eyes were no longer crossed, the lenses of his glasses were much thinner, and he was sitting at the table using silverware and eating the same food as everyone else. He still had a little drag to his right foot, but he walked well and used his right hand and arm effectively. I still hear from both him and his mother. He has a law degree and practices in Brussels.

Impossible Cases

Clearly, CranioSacral Therapy was able to accomplish things that were totally unexpected. I was not always able to predict what the outcome of its application might be, but I felt very strongly that it was essentially risk-free. I continue to think it is always worthwhile to try it and see what happens — especially in "hopeless" cases.

Let me share with you a few more instances in which CranioSacral Therapy accomplished "the impossible." One was a fourteen-year-old boy who had been retarded since he suffered *meningitis* at age five. His uncle was a surgeon, and he had seen to it that the boy had every possible treatment that might be helpful — starting from when he had the *meningitis* and continuing until his mother brought him to me at age fourteen. I treated him twice-weekly for about four months. The first noticeable result was that soon he no longer needed a nap after school every day. Then his speech hesitation improved. Next, the tutor who had been working with him for about two years to help him get a high-school diploma suggested that private tutoring would no longer be necessary. His parents had him retested by the same psychologist who had done his pretreatment evaluation. His IQ had gone up twenty points. He graduated from high school with a strong "B" average. He went on to junior college and got an associate's degree in medical technology. For the past ten years he has been the general manager of a clinical laboratory in a large city. He has about one hundred employees to keep busy. So much for the permanency of mental retardation.

I believe that CranioSacral Therapy was able to improve both the blood supply to his brain and the flow of his *cerebrospinal fluid*. His retardation was probably due to a chronic deficiency of oxygen and nutrients to his brain. He too stays in touch with me and comes to Florida about once a year for a "tune-up" treatment.

Another impossible case was a three-year-old boy who had never talked. He had been to neurologists and speech pathologists. The outlook given to the parents was very glum. No one knew what was wrong or gave any hope of his learning to talk. I treated the boy once during a class I was teaching in California. I found and corrected a severe restriction of the *craniosacral system* overlying one of the speech centers *(planum temporale)* on the left side of his head. The father called me at my hotel the next morning and told me his son had spoken his first words in the car on the way home. Today the boy is fine and, if anything, it is difficult to get him to stop talking.

*   *   *

These are not miracles. They are examples of what can happen if you treat a physiological system, the existence of which has not been previously acknowledged or understood.

The Upledger Institute and The Upledger Foundation

I left Michigan State University in 1983 in order to develop a prototype holistic health center for a private, nonprofit corporation. It was during this time I became aware that, while I was using a wide variety of treatment modalities, I kept returning to CranioSacral Therapy as my mainstay. In 1985 I decided to stop working against that which the fates had planned for me, and we opened The Upledger Institute. In 1987 we established our Upledger Foundation. Since the birth of these two organizations we have learned something from each of the thousands of patients we have seen. In addition, we have trained over fifty thousand practitioners worldwide from a wide variety of healthcare professions in the basic philosophy and techniques of CranioSacral Therapy. Over half of these introductory students have gone on to study intermediate and advanced levels of CranioSacral Therapy.

As our experience broadens and deepens, so our knowledge expands. Since 1985 we have come a long way and are forever grateful to all the patients who have been our teachers. It has become a major tenet in the philosophy of CranioSacral Therapy that if a treatment session does not teach the therapist something, that session has not been a true success.

2

The Offspring of CranioSacral Therapy

Like a chain reaction, the development of CranioSacral Therapy led us to several new concepts about how biological systems work and to new methods of working with the health of human beings and other vertebrates.

The purpose of this chapter is to examine these "offspring" of CranioSacral Therapy. Some of the more significant of these new concepts and practices are: *energy cysts*, tissue memory, SomatoEmotional Release®, Therapeutic Imagery and Dialogue, the Inner Physician, tissue and cellular consciousness, body-mind-spirit integration, the physical aspects of emotional energy, the contagion of emotion and attitude, the retention effects of drugs over a lifetime, the high level of consciousness function of the *fetus* and of the newborn, and the need to complete biological processes that have been initiated.

Energy Cysts and the Significance Detector

We hit upon the concept of *energy cysts* as follows. Dr. Karni, the biophysicist whom I mentioned in the previous chapter, was working with me making bioelectric measurements on patients as I treated them. He observed that I, in a way I was unconscious of, often found a way to help a patient into a position that alleviated pain lingering from old injuries. This happened routinely as a part of my treatment process. Dr. Karni pointed out to me that the electrical potential of the patient's body dropped abruptly when these positions of "ease" were attained. I then realized that the rhythmical activity of the *craniosacral system* stopped very abruptly at those moments. These two phenomena occurred at precisely the same time.

Then we noted that if we kept the patient in that position long enough, the *craniosacral rhythm* would begin again. At the same time, the baseline of electrical potential would rise about half the distance it had dropped; it would be smoother. When we held the patient's body position long enough for these two observed changes to run their courses and for stabilization to occur, we found that the patient's symptoms would be permanently improved, if not totally gone.

I also noted with my hands that heat radiated from a specific area of the patient's body while his/her body was in the "position of ease." We decided to record these heat releases with a thermograph, an instrument that measures and depicts on a screen the temperature of the skin as it changes. This confirmed that the specific body position that produced the other phenomena we had observed also produced the release of heat. The change in local skin temperature was most often about three or four degrees Fahrenheit. The release of heat ended about the same time that the electrical potential and the *craniosacral rhythm* returned to what we called "physiological normal." More often than not, the heat release occurred on an area of skin that the patient identified as the place where the original trauma had occurred—that is, where some external force had struck the body or where the body had landed in a fall. We interpreted the measurable release of heat from the point of injury as a release of energy. We called the storage of this energy in the body an *"energy cyst."*

We came to think of the stored energy as a cyst for the following reason: The energy of the injury penetrated the body a specific distance, determined by the thickness or density of the tissues in relationship to the force of the injury's impact. If for some reason the patient's body was unable to dissipate the force or energy of injury, it would localize and compact this foreign energy into the smallest possible space. We called this compaction the *energy cyst.* We theorized that this was the body's method of minimizing the effect of this foreign energy upon the nearby tissues.

We called the interruption of *craniosacral system* rhythm, when the body went into the position of ease, the Significance Detector, as I mentioned before. The Significance Detector was confirmed by the electrical changes and the recorded heat release. We decided it was the patient's body tissues that led me to the proper position in which the injury occurred.

We soon understood that these *energy cysts* and tissue memories were not limited to physical phenomena. Quite often we saw that the release of an *energy cyst* from a patient's body was accompanied by the re-experiencing of an emotion that was related to the injury. For example, a patient injured in an automobile accident might recall and relive the fear and frustration experienced as he saw the accident coming and was powerless to prevent it. He might have seen the accident coming just before his head hit the windshield. During therapy, while the *energy cyst* was being released from the head, and the long-standing post-traumatic head pain was subsiding, he might spontaneously relive and release the emotional component of the accident. Once all of this physical and emotional releasing had occurred, the symptoms would be permanently gone. I call this phenomenon "SomatoEmotional Release" (SER).

SomatoEmotional Release®:
A Puzzle Solved and a Process Named

The concept of SomatoEmotional Release was placed before me by three factors coming together. The first factor was the work with Dr. Karni, which led us to understand that foreign energy can be retained in "cystic" form for many years, causing symptoms during that time. The second factor was our work with *autistic* children. The third factor involved an experience with a female patient that I will describe shortly.

My work with *autistic* children was going on concurrently with the *energy cyst* work I was doing with Dr. Karni. We were seeing these children change for the better, emotionally and behaviorally, when we helped them move into body positions that facilitated emotional release and reorganization. All these children needed was for us to place our hands on them in a loving way. Then, as we administered CranioSacral Therapy and their bodies began to trust us, they went into body positions that were dictated by their own tissues. In these positions they released energy that we could feel, and their *craniosacral rhythm* stopped until the release was complete.

We did not make measurements on these children because to do so would have required taking them about fifty miles away from their school to our university laboratories. This was simply not feasible at the time for many reasons. We did, however, do some *thermographic* studies. We observed that when they were in a body position that allowed for the release of the emotional energies, the skin temperature of their hands usually moved towards normal. The rise in hand temperature was often four or five degrees Fahrenheit. I guessed that this

hand warming signified a reduction of stress (probably physiological and emotional) involving the whole body as com-
pared to *energy cysts,* which are very localized. Somato-
Emotional Release involves the whole body.

The release of emotion in these children was a real puzzle
for me. How could body position, dictated by the *autistic* child
and facilitated by the therapist, cause release of pathological
emotions? I still don't know quite how it works, but my experience with a certain female patient certainly brought all the
pieces together.

She was a thirty-six-year-old divorced woman working in
the state school system as a superintendent in the special-education division. She was referred to me for biomechanical consultation by the department of psychiatry. She had been in psy-
chiatric treatment for over five years. Her complaints were
severe headaches and worse low-back pain. Both problems
were constant at some level, and, when they worsened, she
would be unable to work for a day or two at a time. Her headaches had not been classified as migraines. There was no evi-
dence of ruptured or "slipped" discs in her low back. She had
not had a single totally pain-free day since her *hysterectomy*
at age twenty-eight. The surgery had been done at her request.
There was no tumor. She was childless. Today this type of elective surgery at so young an age would not be performed, but
in the 1960s a woman could usually get a *hysterectomy* if she
asked for it.

During our first treatment session I released the muscles at
the base of her skull, upper neck and back. I then released her
lower spinal *(lumbar)* vertebrae as well as her *left sacroiliac.*
She was pain-free for the first time in years. I suggested that
she return for more treatment if the pain came back. About a
week later she called for an appointment because the pains,

both head and low back, were returning, though they were not too bad as yet. I saw her again about a week after her call. Her pains were back in full force by that time. I used the same treatment as in our first session. This time there was no relief. When I finished her rather routine biomechanical treatment, she began to yell at me for not trying. She told me that I must hate women, that I had no right to be a doctor, and so on. I just listened and told her I was sorry she wasn't feeling better. She calmed down very quickly and asked for another appointment in a week. I obliged her. Then I called her psychotherapist to report her outburst and to get some history.

It seems the reason for her elective *hysterectomy* was that her husband had threatened to end their marriage if she didn't do something about her "terrible" PMS *(premenstrual syndrome)*, which was making his life unbearable. He first suggested the *hysterectomy*, then he insisted upon it. She gave in, resigned herself to remaining childless, and had the surgery. She chose a *vaginal hysterectomy* in order to avoid an abdominal scar, which would have been offensive to her husband. About a year after the *hysterectomy* he filed for divorce and they separated. She had not had a meaningful relationship since that time.

Her therapist reported that she was extremely angry at men in general—a fact to which I could now testify—and had been suffering headaches and low-back pain since age twenty-eight. She wound up in psychotherapy because all else had failed. The psychotherapist told me that her progress in dealing with her anger was poor and that she had not been able to gain any help with the pains—hence the referral for biomechanics evaluation and treatment. With this background information somewhat digested, I felt a lot of compassion for this woman when she came in for the next appointment. She was polite and apologized a little for her outburst the last time I had seen her. She laid down on her back on the treatment table. To her left, within arm's reach, was a chair upon which she placed a rather large and heavy purse. I had a student with me during this session as part of his preceptorship. I began by examining her low back. I was on her left with my right hand under her *left sacroiliac*. With my left hand I brought her left leg to a position wherein the thigh was vertical, pointing towards the ceiling, and the knee was bent at about a ninety-degree angle. I was inducing slight movements in the knee through the thigh in order to move the *left ileum (pelvic bone)* and test the degree of motion or tightness of her *left sacroiliac*.

All was going well, and I felt that I was beginning to relieve some of the restriction of motion in this *sacroiliac joint*. My student was standing across the table from me as I was explaining what I was doing. Suddenly I felt a blow to the back of my head. She had hit me with her purse! She immediately apologized, saying it was not me she was angry with, it was the surgical resident who leaned on her knee during her operation and caused her back problem. I realized immediately that the position in which I had put her leg was the same position her leg would have been in during her *vaginal hysterectomy*. During this surgery both legs would be up in stirrups, and it would be quite usual for the surgical resident to be standing to one side with his hand(s) upon her knee, perhaps leaning on it to some degree. Since her whole body was anesthetized (she had a general anesthetic) during this surgery, it wouldn't have taken much force to strain a *sacroiliac joint*. The muscles that ordinarily protect against such strains are rendered helpless by the drugs used. I explained to her that residents usually work twelve or more hours a day. I assured her that he had meant her no harm and that he was probably just very tired. She had no reason to be angry with him. She didn't accept my attempt at peace-making. She was sure that he had done this damage to her back on purpose. I then explained that if she kept her anger at him, her back couldn't get well. I reminded her that after our first session she was pain-free in her back for almost a week. I told her that if she let go of her anger, her back pain could disappear. She said, quite simply, "Okay."

As she said this I felt heat come out of her *sacroiliac,* then it relaxed and became very supple. She smiled, just momentarily. During that brief moment I thought that the treatment session was finished. Not so. Something inside of her did not want the session to end. It was as though she knew we were on the right track and that we should keep going while we were on a roll. Her head went back into *hyperextension* (backward bending). Neither my student nor I were at the end of the table where her head was located. Her upper back arched so that her shoulders were off the tabletop. My student was afraid that she was having a *seizure.* I recognized that the *hyperextension* of the head, neck and upper back was reminiscent of the position a patient is put in when the anesthesiologist is placing a breathing tube down the patient's throat.

I went to the head end of the table. We moved her body so that the table would not interfere with the backward bending of her head and neck. I supported her neck and the back of her head in as caring and gentle a way as I could. She was choking and gurgling as though the breathing tube was being passed. I began to whisper in her ear that it was all going very well and she could relax. She did. Then I asked her if she could describe to me what was going on. I told her she should stay in the experience, but that part of her could act as an observer and describe to me what she was seeing and hearing.

She described the *intubation* first. She then described a conversation between the surgeon and the anesthesiologist; both were men. The surgeon said it was strange that a woman twenty-eight years of age who had no children should request an elective *hysterectomy* when there was no real pathological problem that required it. He said it was really not his concern, however, and it was her choice. She became a little angry at his expressed lack of concern. Then the anesthesiologist quipped that it was okay because she was "losing the baby carriage but keeping the playpen." In other words, perhaps all she wanted was foolproof birth control.

She became furious at the anesthesiologist. I tried to explain that anesthesiologists and, perhaps a bit less so, surgeons develop a defense mechanism for their own sanity, which keeps them from feeling compassion for their patients to some extent. The anesthesia people seem to be particularly detached because they routinely have to take patients towards death's door and then keep them in limbo, preventing them from passing through the door, until the surgeon has finished his work. Then they have to revive these injured patients who have been mutilated, perhaps artfully, but nonetheless cut up. It is hard to take this risk with patients' lives day after day without remaining detached.

In this case the surgeon expressed a bit of compassion and then denied it. The anesthesiologist went a step further and made light of the situation. Neither doctor knew the reason for the elective *hysterectomy* nor the emotional baggage carried with it. I explained all of this to her while she was suspended in the re-experiencing of the surgical setting. She would not accept any such excuses. She was angry with the surgeon and furious with the anesthesiologist—the surgeon for his lack of compassion and the anesthesiologist for his lack of respect.

Then, perhaps inspired by the success with anger discharge a few minutes earlier, I simply said that if she remained angry her head would continue to hurt. If she would release the anger and fury, she could rid herself of the pain. She said, "Okay." Her neck softened, heat came out, her skull moved easily on her neck, and her pain left. She then came back to the here and now, smiling, with no pain. This time I asked her to come back in a week. My student rather emphatically requested that he too be invited to her next appointment.

When she returned she reported that she had no pain, but was rather nervous and agitated. She was quick to lose her temper and impatient with interruptions in her regular schedule. She also informed me that she had not seen her psychotherapist since our first visit.

By pre-arrangement with my student, as soon as she lay down on the treatment table on her back, he picked up her right leg and I her left. We gently, but rather quickly, positioned her legs in the positions they would have been in during the *vaginal hysterectomy*. She immediately went to a state of consciousness wherein she was back on the surgical table.

She picked up the experience where she had left it the last time. She had no problem being in the experience and describing as an observer what was happening. During this session I found that I could converse rather freely with her "observer" aspect. She gave a very detailed description of the surgical procedure, both in terms of how it felt to her and how she saw it from a station somewhat above her body. She described the cutting, the tugging and pulling, the *electrocautery* to control bleeding, the final delivery of her *uterus* through her *vaginal canal,* and the placement of the removed organ in a metal basin to be sent to the pathology laboratory for microscopic examination.

Once the *uterus* was removed, the surgeon stepped aside and told the surgical resident to "close the vaginal cuff" located high up in the vagina. This meant that the resident was to sew the opening closed. This sewing is called *"suturing,"* and the thread is called *"suture."* The patient felt the resident putting nine separate *suture*s into this vaginal cuff. She felt the needle piercing her tissue; she felt the *suture* sliding through the holes that were made by the needle; and she felt the squeezing of the tissues as the *sutures* were pulled snug and the knots tied. I have been involved in enough of these surgeries to feel confident that her descriptions were authentic. Even though she was fully anesthetized and supposedly oblivious to what was going on, some part of her was sensing and recording these events in a memory bank somewhere in her brain. Today I believe they were also recorded in some of her body tissues besides the brain, and perhaps outside of her *nervous system* entirely.

In any case, when the resident was through he stepped away, and the surgeon came back to review the resident's work. (Our patient commented that while the resident was sewing her up, the surgeon had been off to the side discussing plans for a Sunday afternoon barbecue. He was inviting the nurse and her husband to come to the party.) Upon his return to the operative site, the surgeon quickly looked at the resident's work and began to berate the resident for doing "such a sloppy job." He said he wanted to make the resident remove the *suture*s and do the thing over again, but there was no time. Once again, our patient was very angry at the surgeon's attitude and the lack of caring that seemed prevalent in the whole situation.

I explained that residents were generally treated as "second-class citizens," and that part of the surgeon's job was to decimate the resident's ego in order to keep him in a subservient position throughout his years of surgical training. During these years residents work ungodly hours, are tremendously underpaid, and have to serve the certified surgeon's whims and fancies as well as do their regular work. Surgeons keep residents in these roles doing the "skut" work by continually reminding them that they hardly ever do anything right.

Once again, our patient refused to let go of her anger based on this explanation, so I simply said that if she continued to keep the anger she would be agitated, quick-tempered, unhappy, etc., probably for the rest of her life. I asked her to release this anger. She said, "Okay," and as she did we could feel her whole body relax. She smiled, and the treatment was over. She did not return to psychotherapy, nor did she return to me as a patient; however, she did guest-lecture to my class every quarter for about three years. She described her experience and tried to impress upon the students how important it is to watch what they are saying, even when the patient is fully anesthetized. I added that they should be careful even when the patient is in a coma or is a newborn who supposedly doesn't know what those around them are talking about.

I put these three experiences together: 1) the energy cyst release work with Dr. Karni; 2) the *autistic* children's improvements due to changes in body positions; and 3) the placing of the patient's body back into the position she was in during her surgery, which resulted in her conscious recall of the events, emotions and procedures that occurred under general anesthesia. It was apparent that there was a link between body position, tissue memory and emotional release. It seemed as though body tissues could contain emotion and release it under the appropriate circumstances. It was clear that pain in body tissues could be caused by emotional energies locked into them, as well as by traumatic forces retained by them; that *energy cysts* retain both emotional energy and the energy of the injury; and that whole bodies retain emotions in the form of energy.

At this point I needed a name for the process of emotional release we had witnessed in all these circumstances, one that would distinguish such release from "psychosomatic" phenomena where the mind is the cause of bodily symptoms. I also needed a name for the treatment itself that facilitated the release. I decided upon "SomatoEmotional Release" (SER). "Somato" is the combining form of the Greek word "soma," which means body. We were using the body to effect emotional release. When the emotional and/or traumatic energies were well localized, we called this "Energy Cyst Release."

More Names:
Inner Physician; Therapeutic Imagery and Dialogue

Once I had found the name SomatoEmotional Release, I realized that there were still other aspects of the process I needed terms for. In working with the woman who had undergone the *hysterectomy*, I had conversed with a separated part of her self that stood in observation of the process she was going through. In other cases, such a separated part of a patient had proven to be quite knowledgeable about the patient's ailment and symptoms. I therefore came up with the term "Inner Physician" for the entity conversed with, and the phrase "Therapeutic Imagery and Dialogue" for the process of conversing with it. (What "imagery" has to do with it will become clear in a moment.)

Once I had these terms in hand, the concepts developed in very rapid fashion. In fact, it became clear that by connecting very deeply with a patient while doing CranioSacral Therapy, it was possible in most cases to solicit contact with the patient's Inner Physician. It also became clear that the Inner Physician could take any form the patient could imagine—an image, a voice or a feeling. Usually, once the image of the Inner Physician appeared, it was ready to dialogue with me and answer questions about the underlying causes of the patient's health problems and what could be done to resolve them. It also became clear that when the conversation with the Inner Physician was authentic, the *craniosacral rhythm* went into a holding mode. This was the same Significance Detector that signaled the therapeutic position for an Energy Cyst Release and the position of release for the whole-body emotional changes that occurred with *autistic* children.

When an image of the patient's Inner Physician presented itself to the patient, the Significance Detector could usually be relied upon to let us know whether this image was authentic. If an image presented itself without the Significance Detector's verification, it often meant, we discovered, that some part of the patient's being was playing a game with us. What sort of game? Perhaps to test our skills or our good will or our sincerity before entrusting us with the real truth. But when the Significance Detector appeared, it invariably indicated authenticity, and it became possible to gain information about almost anything that was happening in the patient's being.

A Few Examples
The Inner Physician

A few case histories seem in order at this point. The first is a good illustration of the extraordinary usefulness of the Inner Physician.

A woman in her late fifties who was a student of CranioSacral Therapy, and a person therefore well-versed in its potential uses, came to see me. She had just received pathology lab results reporting a highly invasive type of cancer in her left breast that had spread to her left *axilla* (armpit). There was no *metastasis* apparent in the lungs or brain, both favorite places for these particular tumors to establish themselves. She was scheduled for surgery in ten days; she wanted to see me before then. We scheduled four appointments for the week preceding her surgery.

During the first session both she and I established a very authentic connection with her Inner Physician. Her Inner Physician informed us that the reason for the occurrence of the breast cancer was to call her attention to the fact that she was neglecting and actually resenting her role as wife and mother. She was successful in her career, but was becoming dominant and inconsiderate of her husband and children. Even though the children were grown, they still needed her.

Previously she had developed *endometriosis* (a female disease), which had been treated by *hysterectomy* about ten years before. Her Inner Physician said that the *endometriosis* was also an attempt to draw her attention to her being female, but that the removal of her *uterus* had further separated her from her role as wife and mother.

Further dialogue revealed the reason she was trying to divorce herself from being a woman. She had been raped in her early adolescence, and this caused her to wish she was not female. All of this came out in about a forty-five minute session, during which I was treating her *craniosacral system* as I dialogued with her. The CranioSacral Therapy seemed to facilitate the rest of the process, in this case the search for an underlying reason for the cancer. I also established a dialogue with the malignant tissues and connected to the tumors with my hands. I asked the tumors if they wanted her dead. The reply was "not necessarily." She simply needed to accept and appreciate her role as a woman. We then released the physical and emotional energies that were still present from the rape that had happened over forty years before. This done, I asked her to consider what we had come up with and see how she felt about the whole thing.

The next day she agreed that she had resented her womanhood for most of her life. In order to stay alive, she was willing to be the wife and mother that part of her was demanding she be. During this session we focused upon converting the malignant cells to benign cells. This was the way she wanted to do it.

We held long dialogues with her Inner Physician and the malignant cells, and did hands-on work with her *craniosacral system*. All of this was aimed at releasing restrictions in her *craniosacral system*, ironing out the details of the changes it would be necessary to make in the way she was living her life, and discovering how the malignant cells might become benign.

At her third appointment there wasn't much new to do—just work further with details, fine-tune the *craniosacral system*, and reassure her. She felt confident. We decided that we could cancel her fourth (and last) scheduled appointment. She went home, which was across the country. She called me the following Monday. She had postponed her surgery against the surgeon's advice. He was very emphatic that she should have a radical mastectomy with removal of the *lymph nodes* in the *axilla*. The tumors had not changed in size. Her husband and children wanted her to go through with the surgery. Her husband became angry at her postponement and told her he would leave her if she didn't go through with the surgery.

She was a bit confused, but as we talked she decided to honor the needs of her husband and children. She had the surgery on Thursday of that week. Three large tumors were found in the breast that was removed, and twenty *lymph nodes* were removed from her *axilla*. *None of these tumors or* lymph nodes *showed any sign of malignancy!*

The Significance Detector and the Inner Physician

The next case I will describe is that of a four-month-old baby boy who was as floppy as a rag doll. It was in France, and the CranioSacral Therapist who had been working with him for a few weeks brought him in just for my evaluation. The parents did not speak English, and the baby had never been exposed to the English language in his young life. I decided to try to communicate with this four-month-old "floppy baby" anyway. The child had been born in a local French hospital. There were forty French therapists in my class. I was teaching through an interpreter. I put my hands on the baby as he lay on the table. He was very flaccid, and his cry was very weak. The French doctors had no idea what had gone wrong. He was born "floppy" and had not progressed much in the four months since his birth.

I decided to see if the Inner Physician would communicate with me *via* the *craniosacral system*. I requested aloud in English that the *craniosacral rhythm* stop if the answer to a question was "yes" and not stop if the answer was "no." The rhythm stopped for about ten seconds. I took this as an indication that I was being understood. I then asked if it was possible during this session for the rhythm to stop only in response to my questions and not for other reasons, such as body position, etc. The rhythm stopped again. I was feeling more confident. I proceeded.

First I asked if there was any structural damage or deficit in the brain. The answer was "no." Then I asked if it was possible to do something to get the brain to start working normally. The answer was "yes." I asked if it was a problem that occurred after delivery? "No." Was it a problem that occurred during delivery? "No." Was it something that occurred while in the *uterus*? "Yes."

With yes-no answers, I pinned the time down to something that happened during the second week of the fourth month of pregnancy. I then established that it was not due to any viral or bacterial infection of either mother or *fetus*. Ultimately, I determined that the problem was due to a toxin that was inhaled by the mother; it was not medicine, food, etc. We found that it was due to the inhalation of organic solvents over a period of about two-and-a-half hours while cleaning the grease off an antique automobile engine for her husband. He liked to rebuild antique cars and sell them. She inhaled the organic solvent fumes and they got to the *fetus via* the *placenta* and *umbilical cord*. The fetal body was able to handle everything except the toxic effect on the brain. The toxic molecules interrupted the development of function of the motor control area of the brain. The parts were all there; they just needed to be jump-started.

I asked many particulars about what I should do. I was told to pump up the action of the paired *parietal bones* that form a large part of the roof of the skull, and to pass a lot of my energy through the brain from the back of the skull to the front. I did what I understood to be correct, checking in frequently with the *craniosacral rhythm* to find out if I was doing it right. The whole process took less than an hour. As I was doing the treatment suggested by the Inner Physician, the baby began to move his arms and legs, to shift his trunk around, and finally to lift his head by himself.

When I finished, the mother took the baby in her arms. She wept in gratitude and the baby cried loudly as he wiggled and squirmed vigorously. I would hesitate to tell this story except that I had forty-four French therapists as witnesses.

About five years later I was teaching in France and my interpreter asked me if I remembered this child. I did. He told me that the boy's development had been normal and that he was now in preschool. His parents sent their love.

The Inner Physician and Drug Addiction

Another case is that of a middle-aged man who had been in a severe automobile accident about fifteen years before I saw him. He was hospitalized for about six weeks while bone grafts were done and a multitude of fractures healed. During his hospital stay he became addicted to morphine. When he was released he was put on less potent pain killers that did not satisfy his craving. He was single without family responsibilities, so he turned to street drugs. Soon he had traded a morphine addiction for a heroine addiction.

Then he fell in love. He forced himself to stop using heroine or any other narcotic drugs. He married and had two children. I had successfully treated his children, the elder for a bite problem in order to avoid orthodontics, and the younger for a learning disability involving reading and the formation of words into phrases and sentences as he spoke.

Both children turned out well, so he decided to confide the story of his narcotic addiction. He had been clean for about twelve years, but every day he still had the desire to "shoot up." Could I help him? I said I didn't know where we would go, but I was willing to try. We did CranioSacral Therapy, which led to multiple Energy Cyst Releases and then to Somato-Emotional Releases that were very powerful. Ultimately, his Inner Physician came forward. It described to me that the residue of both morphine and heroine still remained in his body. As long as that was present he would have drug cravings. The Inner Physician led me to the pockets of drug residue. I mobilized the fluid movement through the areas and passed energy through them.

In about the fourth session I received word from his Inner Physician that the clearing task was complete. The next day the patient came in for his appointment very happy. He said that for the first time since his hospitalization he awakened in the morning with no desire for any morphine or heroine. That was several years ago. He stays in close touch with me because he has been studying CranioSacral Therapy for the past several years. He says that the cravings have never returned.

But What Is It?

By now you must understand that the Inner Physician can be helpful in a wide variety of situations. At this time in my practice I have come to rely upon it and trust it completely. What exactly the Inner Physician *is* doesn't matter to me. It works. My *entrée* to it is through the *craniosacral system*. I have gone from being a rather hard-line scientific-type physician to one who says that if it works I'll use it; I don't have to understand it first. At present I believe that CranioSacral Therapy and its progeny are in the business of reuniting the body, mind and spirit into a whole being again. We have separated the whole person into smaller and smaller parts in an attempt to understand more about how it all works. That is okay, but we have not focused on putting all these parts back into a contextual whole. It is time to view the whole patient. CranioSacral Therapy does that.

Emotions Can Be Contagious

Experience has shown us that *fetuses* and newborns receive many of the emotions of their parents, especially of the mother while the baby is still in the womb. Fearful mothers often implant their fears into the *fetus*, and a fearful baby is delivered for no apparent reason. It would seem that emotions such as fear, guilt, anger, etc., are contagious to the unborn child; so are happiness, joy, serenity, and so on. Emotions can be released using our techniques when it seems desirable. The Inner Physician can tell you where they come from. Awareness of attitude and feelings on the part of the parents is important for the infant during a pregnancy. If a conscious effort to encourage positive emotions is made, positive emotions will, by contagion, enter the child. Children are very aware of the emotional environment in which they live. This would seem to be the case from conception through the preschool years.

Completion of the Biological Process

There is another offspring of CranioSacral Therapy I have dubbed "Completion of Biological Process." This concept and the techniques that are used in relation to it came from the Inner Physicians of five women who presented with similar problems over a period of two months. Their biological clocks were ticking. They were all between thirty-five and forty years of age and had no children; they were all professionals enjoying their various careers; and they were all experiencing similar inner conflicts about having a child before it was too late. There was a certain desperation about the situation for all of them. When this desperation gained the upper hand, each of them was tempted to go to a sperm bank, marry the first man who said "yes" to their proposal, or simply become pregnant by almost any man who would be a knowing or unknowing sperm donor. During more rational days, these women would be concerned about making at least a partial sacrifice of their careers to motherhood.

The drive to be a mother is a very powerful one. I asked the first woman's Inner Physician if there might be an effective method of calming the drive without delivering a baby. The suggestion came from her Inner Physician to guide her through an imaginary pregnancy and delivery. The more details imagined, the more effective the result would be.

I was experienced in obstetrics, so I could talk this first woman through the process. I had her select a father and then image the conception, the implantation, and the fetal development month by month. I talked her through the typical discomforts of pregnancy, always offering alternatives so that it was her pregnancy, not my concept of her pregnancy. Then we imaged through a labor and delivery. I helped make this process as comfortable as possible by minimizing labor pains, suggesting that forceps were not necessary, and so on. When the baby was born, she immediately bonded with her child's image; she nursed it, stayed with it, and loved it for several minutes. Then, when she was ready, she let the baby go off into the cosmos. She felt it was a spiritual birth, and she released the spirit of the child when it was completed. Her Inner Physician approved of the process. I kept in touch with this woman for a few months. Her strong drive to have a child seemed satisfied. She continued in her career and was no longer desperate or even concerned to enter the ranks of motherhood.

As fate seems to plans things, four more women, very similar to this first one, came to me about this time. All of them went through similar processes with me as their guide. All four continued their careers without becoming mothers. Their drive to become mothers was released. In each case the work was completed while I was working with my hands through the *craniosacral system*.

A concept developed for me as I worked with these women. It was that the first ovulation triggers a coded process that is supposed to go to completion. If the process is thwarted for any reason, it drives the woman to want to have a child "before it is too late." She does not have to go through a real pregnancy and delivery, however, to complete the process; it can be satisfied by an *imaged* one.

This approach can be applied to a variety of incomplete biological processes, and may be very helpful in the resolution of several kinds of internal conflicts. Since the time I worked with these women, I have used it for miscarriages and abortions by imaging the completion of the pregnancy and the delivery of the baby. When we do this, residual guilt and/or conflict resolves. Several fertility problems have also been solved by completing the incomplete pregnancy through imaging.

3

The Guiding Principles of CranioSacral Therapy

For CranioSacral Therapy and its offspring to work properly, it is required that the practitioner have trust in the fact that within each patient lies the information necessary to understand the underlying causes for health problems and what must be done to resolve them. It thus becomes the responsibility and goal of the CranioSacral Therapist from the beginning to establish a working rapport with this well of information and understanding. It is this inner wisdom that makes the appearance of the Inner Physician possible.

In order to develop this high-quality rapport, the therapist must impart to the nonconscious inner wisdom of the patient that his or her intentions are to help deal with primary problems, not to mask core issues by offering symptomatic relief. Deep problems must be defined and resolved.

The Inner Physician knows this and will not settle for less. If one set of symptoms is "cured" but a deeper problem is not resolved, this deeper problem may find another set of symptoms to present. It is as though the symptoms are a call for help from deep inside the patient. Core problems may be physical, emotional and/or spiritual. The CranioSacral Therapist must establish a relationship with the Inner Physician in order to help the patient get to this problem. When the deeper problem is resolved, the symptoms dissolve with perhaps just a little help from the therapist.

I do not want to lead you to believe that all symptoms have deep underlying causes. Some are simply happenings that occur. But in CranioSacral Therapy we believe that every symptom, pain and complaint deserves an investigation to determine whether or not it is the voice of a deeper problem or simply something such as a freak accident, an infection, etc. The Inner Physician knows the answer to this question and will share it willingly with the therapist once a trusting relationship has been established.

*   *   *

The precise principles that guide the development of trust between the Inner Physician and the therapist are as follows:

1. The therapist must focus exclusively on the patient during the session. His/her mind must not be preoccupied with other matters. Inner Physicians can sense distraction—even in therapists with excellent acting skills!

2. The therapist must be open to whatever twists and turns might occur during the session.

3. The therapist's belief system must be suspended.

4. There is no room for judgmental behavior or thoughts on the part of the therapist.

5. The therapist does not heal or cure. The healing is done by the patient using the help and facilitation of the therapist. Symptomatic suppression can be imposed by a

"healing" therapist, but this may only be denying a deeper problem its voice.

6. Initially, CranioSacral Therapy employs a soft, gentle use of the hands to facilitate the self-correction of the *craniosacral system*. Concurrently, this touch is used to convey to the Inner Physician the love, trust and sincere dedication of the therapist. This loving, trusting and dedicated energy is offered without conditions or strings attached in order to facilitate the deepest possible healing.

7. Once trust is established, greater forces may sometimes be required to obtain corrections in the *craniosacral system's* functioning. The therapist may, on occasion, intervene forcefully, always keeping in mind that such action may still be dealing with only superficial restrictions. Correction of these restrictions by the use of external force, even if it brings symptomatic relief, must not be considered deep healing unless the Inner Physician indicates that it is.

8. CranioSacral Therapy always improves fluid movement in all systems throughout the body. By doing this it enhances the supply of nutrients to cells; the removal of toxins and waste products from the tissues; the circulation of immune cells, thus enhancing the body's natural defenses against disease-producing bacteria and viruses; the delivery of fresh blood to organs and tissues; and the movement of *cerebrospinal fluid*. Therefore, there are no situations where it should not be applied, except where the above results are undesirable for some reason.

9. The patient's body will always guide the therapist's hands to the places where they will do the most good. I consider

that this guidance is actually the Inner Physician at work, even before any verbal dialogue has been developed.

10. The CranioSacral Therapist must trust the information received from the patient's body and from the Inner Physician, otherwise the information will stop coming. It is as though the Inner Physician rejects the therapist. In such cases the therapist will be able to do superficial structural work with the *craniosacral system,* but probably will not be able to get to deep problems until the trust is developed.

11. I do not believe that CranioSacral Therapists should think of particular symptoms as always following from the same causes in a one-two fashion. Each patient, and even each occurrence of a symptom in a single patient, is an individual case. Expectations that the same symptom always derives from the same cause can be very misleading, especially when the therapist is relying upon very subtle bodily motion signals as is the case in the use of Cranio-Sacral Therapy. These signals may be merely imagined by the therapist if he/she expects to find them. It is better not to even know the patient's complaint when the body evaluation is done. When I begin a session with a patient I have seen before, I try not to remember what I found out previously; I always evaluate the situation freshly. I may find new developments that might otherwise escape me if I already have a mindset when I re-evaluate. After the initial evaluation for each session, there is plenty of time to integrate your previous findings with the patient's report of changes, new pains, etc.

* * *

I would like to elaborate a bit on principle number 11 at this point.

Our present conventional healthcare system relies a great deal on previous diagnoses and verbal history. We in Cranio-Sacral Therapy operate on the assumption that all you need to know is lying before you on the table at the moment of evaluation. Previous information in general can bias your evaluation. I came to believe this many years ago, before I became involved with CranioSacral Therapy.

In 1966 I was in practice in Clearwater Beach, Florida. One evening I was called upon to make a motel housecall. It was about 9:00 PM when I arrived. A woman was lying on her bed with a very severe headache. Her husband presented me with a letter from a highly reputable medical clinic in the north. The letter stated that his patient suffered from severe migraine headaches. It suggested that the treatment of choice would be fifty to seventy-five milligrams of the powerful synthetic narcotic Demerol by injection in the muscle. I examined her and became very suspicious that she had a brain tumor rather than a migraine headache. I gave her the Demerol for her pain after I completed my examination, which took three or four minutes. The shot helped a little. I tried to convince her husband that he should let me hospitalize her. He finally agreed and we went to the hospital by ambulance. She died during the night. The autopsy revealed that she had malignant brain tumors. Perhaps originally she *had* been a victim of migraines. But failure to re-evaluate each episode afresh may have cost her her life. I decided at the time not to accept previous diagnoses from medical clinics, no matter how reputable.

* * *

Here are some more cases that illustrate the same point.

I recently worked with three patients who would have totally befuddled me had I allowed myself to be influenced by previous experiences. My belief that each patient is different was confirmed in each case. The three cases involved women, all in the thirty- to thirty-five-year-old range. I'll call them patients A, B and C to protect their privacy.

Patient A was an Olympic-class diver who had been forced to drop out of training about three months before seeing me. She suffered from severe *vertigo*, which she informed me was common with high-platform divers such as herself. She had competed in previous Olympics and had high hopes of being a medallist in Atlanta. She had been everywhere, done everything, and now her coach was telling her that she would probably not be able to compete. All the other doctors had sought the cause for the *vertigo* in her head. I evaluated her body and found an old problem in her left knee. She thought I was a little crazy, but this is where I began. I trusted her Inner Physician implicitly. I traced the problem from her knee to her pelvis and low back, which were out of balance because they had to compensate for the knee problem. In the pelvis I found two factors that were important. One was in the muscles that go upwards in her body along the sides of the spine. The second was in the *meningeal membrane (dural tube)* that travels within the spinal canal from the bones at the bottom of the spine, the *sacrum* and *coccyx*, up to the top of the spine and into the skull. The muscles were causing her head to be pulled to the right on top of her neck. During certain movements of her body this could kink the *vertebral artery* that supplies part of the blood to the brain. The unbalanced tension on the *dural tube* was causing the *right temporal bone* to be restricted. There are *two temporal bones*, one on the right and another on the left. These are the bones that house the balance mechanisms in the head. My job was to release the knee so that I could balance the pelvis. This allowed me to release the muscles pulling her head to the right and relieve the kink in the *vertebral artery*. I then had to get into the *craniosacral system* and release the abnormal pull coming from the lower spinal bones so that we could relieve the restrictions in the *right temporal bone*. I was successful with both tasks, but the *craniosacral system* corrected first. When this happened the *vertigo* stopped, but a sense of light-headedness came upon her episodically. In about two weeks I had the *spinal muscles* balanced. The light-headedness stopped. It was clear that she had two problems: one was *vertigo* related to the *craniosacral system*, and the other was a temporary kinking of the right *vertebral artery* related to the imbalance of the *spinal muscles*. Both had to be corrected. Neither would have been corrected had I not found the underlying knee problem. Her Inner Physician let me know this was an injury with no deep emotional or spiritual component. She did compete in the Olympics and took a medal in the high-platform dive.

*   *   *

B is a lady about the same age as A. She came to me because she also had *vertigo*. At times it was so bad that it kept her in bed for a day or two at a time. She had been to several doctors and clinics before coming to me. She heard about what I did with the diver and was encouraged. Her body showed no contributing factors. I found *craniosacral system* problems in her head only, and some problem with an inability of her chest cage to move properly while breathing deeply. I corrected these problems and she experienced temporary relief. During these few initial visits I connected with her Inner Physician and learned there were deep emotional and spiritual problems present. Over a few more treatment sessions I communicated aloud with her Inner Physician. We learned from the dialogue that the vertigo was caused by fear. Her mother had died of breast cancer that developed about five years after the onset of vertigo. B was afraid the same thing would happen to her. Then some very deep anger surfaced. It was focused on her mother for being in bed and being unable to be a mother to her. The mother deserted her by dying. We did SomatoEmotional Release and let go of the anger and fear. That was the end of the vertigo and the restrictions of the chest cage. Had I suspected a knee or pelvis problem in B, as I found in A, we would still be working there, and the vertigo would be continuing.

* * *

C came to me because she was having problems with heart flutters and irregularities. At times her heart rate went up to one hundred and forty per minute, which is in a danger zone no matter what the cause. The accepted average rate for women at rest is about eighty beats per minute. This woman was an athlete, so her normal heart rate had usually been down to about fifty beats per minute. She had been to many doctors, but the problem continued. Surgeons had even removed her *thyroid gland* in the hope of restoring her heart to normal rhythm. Now she had to take *thyroid replacement hormones* the rest of her life. Sometimes a *thyroid gland* gone "crazy" will cause a heart rhythm to go up into the stratosphere. Not so in her case. The surgery did not help. I evaluated her body and, oddly enough, found a left knee problem that had required previous surgery. This knee problem affected the pelvis much as A's knee problem did. However, C's *craniosacral system* was not thrown out of kilter. The muscles that run up next to the spine were affected, however, and the right side of her upper neck was very contracted as a result. The *vertebral artery* was not kinked, but the *vagus nerve* that exits the skull in the midst of these contracted muscles was the problem. The *vagus nerve* on the right side serves, among other things, to exert a governing control upon heart rate. When the *vagus nerve* is compressed, "runaway" heart rhythm can be the result. Releasing the pelvis and the muscles of the neck ended the heart-rhythm problems.

Do you see why each patient needs to be evaluated as though theirs is a case unlike any the therapist has ever seen? Left knees, heart problems, emotions, or a myriad of other things can cause *vertigo*.

Each patient is an individual case. This is a guiding principle in the practice of CranioSacral Therapy. Another guiding principle that must be followed is that the body on the table has all the answers; CranioSacral Therapists just have to tune in, blend with, and listen to that body's wisdom.

Practicing CranioSacral Therapy is a humbling and grounding experience. It cannot be effectively practiced by those who are stroking their own egos by being in a healthcare profession.

4

CranioSacral Therapy
and the Flow of Fluids

In my opinion there are few, if any, times that CranioSacral
Therapy will not prove helpful. It improves fluid motion and
flow at all levels. This is always good except in cases of recent
hemorrhaging, where improving blood flow to the damaged
area could cause the hemorrhaging to start again. Even in
these cases, the cautious and judicious application of Cranio-
Sacral Therapy by a true expert may be helpful.

Let me explain what I mean by fluid motion and flow at
all levels. I think most readers appreciate that good blood flow
to all tissues and organs is essential for good health. Fresh
blood to an organ or tissue brings with it the oxygen and nutrients necessary for the organs and tissues to survive. As this
blood passes through, it delivers its supplies and immediately
collects the by-products and waste materials produced by the
moment-to-moment and day-to-day activities of these organs
and tissues as they serve to keep the whole "you" alive. This
flow of blood also carries with it the blood cells and *antibodies*
that are part of the *immune system*. These *immune cells* and
antibodies protect us from bacteria, viruses and toxic materials that have entered our bodies. The better the blood supply,

the better the components of the *immune system* are able to protect us. Better blood flow means a more efficient policing of your organs and tissues by your *immune system*.

CranioSacral Therapy also enhances the flow of *lymph*. *Lymph* is a yellowish, rather transparent fluid, which is collected from your tissues in all parts of the body. The *lymph* has its own system of collecting vessels that pass through glands called *"lymph nodes."* The *lymphatic fluid* system is an important part of our *immune system*. It collects a lot of toxic by-products from infections as well as from the bacteria and/or viruses that cause infections. *Lymphatic fluid* passes through the *lymph nodes,* which serve as filters to purify the fluid to some extent before it is returned to the *blood system*. Cranio-Sacral Therapy enhances the activity of the *lymphatic system*.

When the blood arrives at the tissues, its load of nutrients, oxygen and *antibodies* are discharged from the blood vessels into a fluid called *interstitial fluid;* this fluid bathes the cells and serves as the vehicle for the movement of all these delivered materials so they can get to the individual cells. These materials are then absorbed by the cells as they are needed. The *antibodies* simply circulate and look for foreign things to neutralize. Some *immune cells* do not necessarily exit the blood vessels unless they receive a chemical or energetic message from the cells indicating their help is required. In this case they exit the blood vessels and attack and kill the unwanted materials. Other *immune cells* routinely patrol outside of blood vessels. *Immune cells* are very expert in recognizing which cells are "self" and which are "non-self." They gain this recognition by knowing the protein markers on the surface of the cells under scrutiny.

The interstitial fluid circulates into the cells where it is then called *"intracellular fluid."* It washes in and out of these cells and passes back into the blood or into the *lymph*. On its way back into these systems it brings with it the waste products; the toxic debris that the *immune cells* have not digested (phagocytized); and the carbon dioxide that has formed as a by-product of the manufacturing of energy within each cell. CranioSacral Therapy enhances the movement of this fluid too.

Clearly, water itself is the universal solvent within the body. Water moves from the heart as it is pumped through the large arteries to the smaller ones. It travels to the capillaries and into the interstitial space between the cells. It backs out of the cells into the interstitial fluid—returning either to the *blood system* or the *lymphatic system*. It goes into the *blood system*. The water then goes through the liver and kidneys, getting rid of the waste it has gathered on its trip. It also picks up *antibodies* from the liver for circulation. Water goes to the spleen to gather more fresh *antibodies* and *immune cells*. It goes to the lungs to get rid of the carbon dioxide it collected and to trade it for oxygen, which it delivers to the tissues. It also goes to the liver, the stomach and the small intestine for collection of nutrients. You can see from this brief description of what water does in our bodies just how important it is that water solutions move about with the least amount of restriction possible—except for those normal control mechanisms that the body uses for efficient regulation.

It stands to reason that any therapy that can enhance fluid movement is a health enhancer; CranioSacral Therapy does just that. Thus, CranioSacral Therapy is generally helpful except in those circumstances where damage to the *vascular system* makes *hemorrhage* a threat.

Allow me to suggest that much of what we call aging occurs because toxic wastes in the cells are not efficiently removed. Enhanced fluid movement can improve toxic waste removal.

Since CranioSacral Therapy moves fluids, it is logical to conclude that it helps the toxic waste removal process. From there it seems reasonable to suggest that CranioSacral Therapy may well slow the aging process.

5

Other Conditions for Which CranioSacral Therapy Has Proven Helpful

Acute Infections

CranioSacral Therapy may help people overcome infections. I have seen it lower fevers rather quickly. Once fever drops, the crisis ends and recovery begins. Given this push from CranioSacral Therapy, recuperation is shorter than it might be otherwise.

Most recently I saw a thirteen-year-old girl who suddenly developed extreme lethargy, fever, swelling and pain in many of her joints, and difficulty staying awake. She had been on a powerful antibiotic for almost two weeks. She had a future appointment scheduled at the Mayo Clinic for consultation because she was responding so poorly. Her family doctor and a consulting infectious-disease specialist were concerned; she seemed to be getting critical. Her mother, whom I had treated years ago subsequent to an auto accident, brought her to my home on a Sunday evening. I worked with her for about an hour and a half. During this session I was able to reduce joint swelling and establish an improved fluid flow. Within twenty-four hours she was much improved. I worked with her again on the following Wednesday. Her condition had remained much improved. Her joint swelling had not returned, her fever was gone, and she was much more awake and alert. I found two areas of restricted motion in her body: one in her left pelvis and the other in her left chest. I suspected these were areas of infection, probably a virus, and I surmised they were probably the last residual areas. Fluid motion was impaired in both areas. I worked to re-establish motion so that the components of her *immune system* could go to work. Her response was good. By the time she went to Mayo about a week later, she was feeling much better. The blood tests confirmed a recent infection by cytomegalovirus (CMV). The *antibody* levels in her blood indicated that the acute infection was now gone. Through mobilization of body fluids, CranioSacral Therapy helped *antibodies* and *immune cells* reach troubled areas. Viruses and bacteria cause swelling and inflammation. This interferes with fluid movement and thus impairs the *immune system*'s "soldiers" from getting to the battlefield. Those viruses and bacteria are smart little rascals.

Chronic Pain Syndromes

CranioSacral Therapy has proven very helpful in a wide array of chronic pain problems. Quite often arthritis, headaches, neuralgias, fibromyalgias, and so on are due to the impairment of fluid flows and an accumulation of toxic materials in the involved areas. This accumulation causes pain and/or inflammation depending upon its components.

Arthritis and Joint Pain

Recently we had occasion to treat a disabled veteran whose knees were very swollen. He was using a wheelchair because bearing weight on his legs was too painful. We worked with him in our intensive-therapy program, which involves about six hours of hands-on CranioSacral Therapy per day for either one or two weeks. He came for the two-week program. At the end of the first week he was out of the wheelchair and was not using any crutches or canes. He had very minimal swelling in his knees. He had been unable to walk without pain for over five years prior to this treatment. Though he initially had trouble believing the results, he now proves to himself and others that he is better by going out for long walks on his own.

Headaches

So many headaches are chronic due to tension, chronic congestion, allergies, migraine (due to improper control of the blood vessels in the head by the nervous system) and hormone imbalances. CranioSacral Therapy is quite effective for all of the above. It finds the reasons for tensions and resolves the underlying causes. It opens drainage systems from the skull and, in this way, alleviates congestion headaches. Sometimes CranioSacral Therapy will, by some unknown mechanism, eliminate allergies. I don't understand how this works, but it does in about forty or fifty percent of patients. CranioSacral Therapy is also very effective in migraines because it identifies the cause of faulty nervous control of the blood vessels and normalizes it.

Many women have *premenstrual syndrome* accompanied by headache. CranioSacral Therapy is very effective in helping to normalize the *hormonal system*. Our success rate here is very high. Usually we find problems in the membrane system in the skull that interfere with the normal functioning of the *pituitary gland*. The *pituitary* is the "master gland" of the *endocrine system*.

Most remarkable is the recent case of a forty-five-year-old

woman with a fifteen-year history of severe headaches related to her menstrual periods. The headaches began after the birth of her second child. She's had no pregnancies since that time. In one treatment session I had with her, I released the *sacrum* and the lower end of her *craniosacral system*. Then some work with her skull released tension in the membranes that relate to the *pituitary gland*. Her Inner Physician let me know that there was nothing more to it. It has been over six months since this single treatment, and she has had no problems since then. She came in recently for what she called a CranioSacral Therapy "tune-up." The six-month tune-up is a good idea. It can release a restriction before its effects magnify and symptoms occur.

Neuralgia

Neuralgia is the term used to indicate nerve pain. It is often caused by an impingement, a "friction," or an inflammatory process related to the nerve. In CranioSacral Therapy we recognize that an impingement can be from a bone pressing on the nerve or from a ligament or spastic muscle. A friction can mean that the nerve is passing through an area of old tissue irritation that has gotten fibrous or accumulated waste products that are either granular or crystalline. The nerve may move back and forth through this area with changes in body position or movements such as walking. The gliding activity by the nerve through the tissues is not smooth, and it sets up a sort of friction that causes nerve pain. The nerve may also cause pain because it is inflamed, perhaps by a virus or because it is passing through an area of inflamed or infected tissue. CranioSacral Therapy is quite effective in resolving all of these situations.

Very recently we had a patient come in whose *neuralgia*

was in the form of *sciatic nerve* pain. This pain was with him most of the time. It began in his lower back and went down his left leg. He had had the pain for thirty-one years. He was very emphatic about the thirty-one years. The pain had motivated him to become a researcher in spinal problems. He had his PhD in biomechanics. He knew that something was irritating the roots of the *sciatic nerve*. This is the big nerve that gets its roots from the lower *spinal cord* and travels down the back of the leg. It is a common complaint that is spoken of as "sciatica." He had tried everything he knew to solve his problem. He heard me speak at a conference and decided to see what CranioSacral Therapy could do for him.

My evaluation suggested that the lower end of the *dural tube* was restricted on the left. This *dural tube restriction* was affecting the *sciatic nerve roots* on the left. They were unable to glide easily through the "sleeves" of *dural membrane* that escorted them to their exits in the spinal column. In addition there was some compressing of the lower spine in a vertical direction when he was standing. This was due to spinal-muscle contracture holding the individual vertebrae together tightly and flattening the discs somewhat. It took me and another therapist about two hours of hands-on work to release the low-back compression and the *dural tube*. Our astonished patient got up from the table with a wide smile saying, "My God." He was pain-free for the first time in thirty-one years. He has stayed pain-free from then until this writing, which is about a month later.

His Inner Physician let us know that he had some deeper issues to deal with that were not related to the back pain. The pain came from an old fall on his back. He will return to work on the deeper issues. We began that process before he left here to return to work to let his fellow researchers know what a *dural tube restriction* can do and how CranioSacral Therapy can release the restriction.

Fibromyalgia

The more modern term *fibromyalgia* includes *myalgia, myositis, fibromyositis,* and so on. There are so many terms for these conditions because they are so poorly understood. Essentially they are chronic contractions of muscles that go on so long and so hard that first they inflame, and then they cause some of the muscle cells to eventually turn into fiber. The *fibrosity* sometimes entraps *nerve receptors* and/or *nerve fibers* causing constant pain. Patients with problems in this category may have a myriad of underlying causes: childhood abuse, postural problems due to structural imbalances, occupational stress, deep anger, guilt, fear, and so on.

The Inner Physician can be extremely helpful in determining the underlying cause of the chronic muscle contracture. How long the contractions have been present and how severe they are, as well as their consistency, will determine where the patients are on the path that goes from painful contracture to inflammatory response to the development of *fibrosity*.

All of this is interesting, but the real healing occurs when the cause of the contractures is known.

In one recent case a fifty-year-old woman lived in constant fear of her father. When she was young her father had instilled the fear by making her go upstairs to her room when his "business associates" came over. His usual mode of operation was to pick her up face-to-face with him and tell her that something very bad could happen to her if she came out of her room and peeked or listened to what was going on. Her *fibromyalgia* developed as she held herself in chronic contracture, especially involving the muscles of her upper back between the shoulder blades and into her neck. With the guidance of her Inner Physician we were able to release the retained fear, which gave her about fifty percent relief from pain.

Now we are in the arduous task of reversing the fibrous changes that have occurred over the years. Restoration of motion along with *craniosacral system* work to reduce the muscle tone caused by the brain and *spinal cord* are helping. Incidentally, she now knows that her father was a "hit man" for the "mob." He is deceased.

Temporomandibular Joint Syndrome (TMJ)

This problem has gained tremendous popularity. It has to do with the joints of the lower jaw becoming dysfunctional for any one or combination of reasons. It causes pain at the side(s) of the face where the joints between the lower jaw bone *(mandible)* and the skull *(temporal bone* on each side) are formed. These are complex joints that involve a disc and gliding motion as well as rotation. Since the *mandible* is a single bone with a joint on both ends, when one side is affected, both joints become involved. In addition to joint pain, it is common for TMJ patients to have neck pain, severe headaches, difficulty concentrating, visual problems and/or ringing in the ears. It is also common for shortness of temper and personality changes to accompany this syndrome.

Surprisingly, the origin of the *temporomandibular joint syndrome* can come from a *craniosacral system* problem that results in an imbalance between the two temporal bones on each side of the head. Other causes include nervous tension that results in tooth grinding and/or jaw clenching. The clenching in particular may cause excessive wear and/or inflammation of the temporomandibular joints and teeth. The problem can also result from whiplash injury of the neck, which causes an uneven pull on the muscles that attach to the *mandible*. It may occur from *malocclusion* that may or may not be primary. *"Malocclusion"* is the term used when the upper and lower teeth do not fit together appropriately.

What must be done with the *temporomandibular joint* patient is to search for the underlying cause of the problem. The list of possible causes is almost endless. Here the *craniosacral system* evaluation and communication with the Inner Physician can be extremely valuable.

As an example, a fifty-nine-year-old woman came to see me about ten years ago. She had dental appliances in her mouth that she was quite addicted to because they gave her some relief from the pain and anxiety. She said she had spent over $20,000 on treatment for her condition. It took several sessions and a lot assurance from me to get her to break her addiction to the appliances.

Ultimately, we found that the jammed *temporal bones*, which I had located earlier, had been there for many years before the *temporomandibular joints* finally gave out and began causing severe joint, head and neck pain, as well as the anxiety I was witnessing. I was able to mobilize the *temporal bones* on several occasions, but the problem always returned. Finally the Inner Physician led us to the source of the problem.

At age sixteen she had disobeyed her mother and gone swimming at a lake in a two-piece bathing suit. While she was coming to the surface next to an anchored raft, a teenage boy dove into the water. Their heads squarely collided. She was hurt, but never told her parents because her "conscience" told her that the "hit" was punishment from God for wearing a two-piece bathing suit. She thought God's punishment was enough; she didn't want more from her mother. When this event was re-experienced and she discharged the energy of the fear and the guilt, she changed. Her *temporal bones* accepted permanent correction. Her addiction to the dental appliances was gone, as were all her related symptoms. I still see her for tune-ups. She is doing very well now at age sixty-nine.

*   *   *

Another very interesting *temporomandibular joint syndrome* patient was the mother of a dentist. He sent her to me with his hands up in the air. She had an appliance to wear when eating, another for sleeping, and another for daytime when not eating. Nothing helped. I evaluated her body and found the primary source of the problem in her right *piriformis muscle* (one of the muscles of the right buttock). She then informed me that she had fainted in her kitchen about a year earlier and had struck the left side of her face on the open oven door as she fell. She had experienced pain in her face ever since. Her son treated it as a *temporomandibular joint* problem. Her *mandible* was indeed very much out of balance; however, no one had been able to get it to respond. I released the right *piriformis muscle* which had been strained when she fell. That was all it took to get the *mandible* permanently balanced and the facial pain to disappear.

Low-Back Problems and Backache

These used to be called *"lumbago."* I don't have a lot to say about this very common problem except that the CranioSacral Therapy approach is an excellent way to find the underlying cause. From there, the problem may be amenable to Cranio-Sacral Therapy and its offspring. It may also require physical therapy, spinal adjustment, postural correction, exercises, acupuncture, etc., depending on the cause. My experience has been that many low-back problems are solvable, but may return if people don't change their couch-potato lifestyles. The *craniosacral system* must be cleared of restriction in order to gain maximal effect from any other treatment process.

Reflex Sympathetic Dystrophy (RSD)

RSD is a very painful condition that results from the *sympathetic nervous system* going out of control for some reason. The *sympathetic nervous system* is a division of the *autonomic nervous system*. It takes over in times of crisis and/or stress. It causes the heart rate and blood pressure to go up. It causes your breathing to speed up and your digestive activities to slow down. It gives you the adrenaline that provides superhuman strength in times of crisis. In other words, it focuses on saving your life when danger is imminent. The *autonomic nervous system* is the involuntary part of your total *nervous system*. It runs your body without you being aware of what it is doing. It keeps you alive.

The pain from RSD is usually very severe. This pain may be localized or may cover the whole body. The "something" that causes the *sympathetic nervous system* to go out of control may be an injury to any of the other divisions of the *nervous system*, an entrapped nerve, an inflammation, a toxicity, or any other circumstance that might feed an abnormal amount of energy into the *sympathetic nervous system*. The sympathetic nerves take the bombardment as long as they can. When the nerves in question can no longer deal with the increased bombardment, they lapse into the RSD state and create great pain. The problem may spread throughout the entire *sympathetic nervous system* and result in total body pain. Conservative medical treatment for this condition is rather ineffective. Surgical removal of involved regions of the *sympathetic nervous system* and/or amputation of the body part may be the treatment of last resort.

We saw one patient whose hand was amputated in an attempt to relieve the intractable pain. Relief was temporary. He came to us because his other hand was becoming painful. The CranioSacral approach has been effective for him thus far.

It is our feeling that the key to helping the RSD patient is the discovery and resolution of the underlying source of excess energy being fed into the *sympathetic nervous system*. Cranio-Sacral Therapy and its offspring seem quite well-suited to finding and treating the underlying causes of RSD and subsequently resolving the pain.

Traumatic Injuries

We treat a multitude of closed-head injuries, spinal cord injuries, "whiplash," and other spinal ligament strains and *nervous system* sequelae due to injuries of body parts. We have variable success depending upon the extent and severity of the injury. We usually do quite well with children who have *seizures* subsequent to their head injuries. Often the *seizures* are totally alleviated without further need for medication. We also get moderate improvement in the movement of paralyzed limbs due to head injuries. We most often see great improvement in intellect and social responsiveness, and a dramatic reduction in temper tantrums. We have seen some remarkable improvement in vision and hearing. Smell and taste often improve very quickly.

We had one woman who lost her short-term memory after an auto accident. MRIs and CT scans were negative, but her memory was so bad that she couldn't remember why she went from one side of a room to the other. I tuned into her *craniosacral system* and her Inner Physician. What I learned was that a lot of excess energy was located in the *hippocampus* region of her brain. This brain structure files things to remember in various regions of the brain, then it retrieves this information upon conscious request. Her Inner Physician informed us that the *hippocampus* was not damaged but disorganized. I was advised how to treat it. I followed the suggestion of the Inner Physician. When the session was over, the patient had her memory back. She was quite ecstatic. I maintained my composure and tried not to show my own surprise. I still get surprised occasionally.

Spinal cord injuries are very unpredictable. I am sure that the earlier we see them the better the results. I can think of three patients who came into our two-week intensive program with paralyzed legs and in wheelchairs. Releasing the *dural tube* enabled them to leave walking. We never know when this kind of seeming "miracle" will occur.

When patients are willing, we'll try our best. It is essentially risk-free treatment and will definitely improve the general health, sense of well-being, and the *nervous system sequelae* as they apply to balance, heart rhythm, breathing, digestion, bowel function, urinary system function, and quite often sexual function.

Whiplash and other *spinal ligament* problems usually respond extremely well to our approach. We treat a large number of these kinds of problems. We expect total healing, and it usually happens.

Degenerative Diseases of the Central Nervous System

We have treated a large number of *multiple sclerosis* patients with only moderate success. We often find a rather significant emotional component along with *multiple sclerosis*. Most often the emotional resistance is such that we have been unable to achieve optimal results with CranioSacral Therapy.

Parkinson's disease, on the other hand, is quite responsive to CranioSacral Therapy. I would speculate that since *cerebrospinal fluid* is now known to circulate between all the cells of the brain, and we enhance the flow of this fluid, we are able to favorably influence the Parkinson's patient.

Until just a few years ago it was thought that the *cerebrospinal fluid* simply bathed the surface of the brain. With the use, however, of radioactive tracers that flow with the *cerebrospinal fluid*, it was observed that when these tracers were injected into the *ventricular system* of the brain, the tracers were distributed throughout the brain substance in a matter of minutes. Since this fluid carries all kinds of "message molecules" that tell cells what to do, and offer intercommunication between cells of different systems, it seems to me that the explanation for our positive results with *Parkinson's disease* may lie in the improvement in *cerebrospinal-fluid* circulation that is achieved through CranioSacral Therapy.

Another recent discovery is that *cerebrospinal fluid* contains molecules that attach to metallic atoms deposited in the brain. Once the metal atoms are attached to the *cerebrospinal-fluid* molecules, they are carried away and excreted from the body. This process is known as *"chelation."* Metal atoms deposited in brain tissue are thought to be causal factors in such problems as *Alzheimer's disease* and senility. The *cerebrospinal fluid* provides a natural *chelation*, and thus the improvement of its circulation through brain tissue may be considered a preventive measure to these brain problems. CranioSacral Therapy enhances *cerebrospinal-fluid* circulation. Therefore, we might consider it a worthy preventive treatment for *Alzheimer's* and senility.

We have also had great success in improving the mental

alertness and brain functioning of elderly citizens who were having difficulty concentrating, putting words together, and so on. I'm sure that we are getting improved circulation of blood, *cerebrospinal fluid, interstitial fluid* and *intracellular fluid,* and that we are clearing accumulated toxic wastes from the brain cells and tissues.

Strokes

We have a lot of experience using CranioSacral Therapy with stroke patients. Strokes usually come in three varieties: the *hemorrhage,* the *embolism* and the *thrombosis.*

The *hemorrhagic stroke* may or may not involve an aneurysm. The aneurysm is a weak spot in an artery that finally gives out and leaks blood into brain tissue. Another form of *hemorrhagic stroke* occurs when the blood pressure goes so high that a blood vessel breaks and blood floods into brain tissue. When free *(extravasated)* blood lies in brain tissue, an extreme irritation occurs, which worsens as the red blood cells deteriorate. Breakdown by-products of blood cells become stronger and stronger irritants as days pass. It helps to wash them out as soon as possible. Therefore, CranioSacral Therapy is indicated as soon as the danger of new or renewed *hemorrhage* passes. The sooner and more efficiently these toxic by-products of blood-cell deterioration are washed away, the less severe the lasting effects of the *hemorrhagic stroke* will be.

The second type of stroke is the *embolism.* This means that an *embolus* (ball) of some type has formed and passed through the *arterial system* to a point where a branching likely occurs and the diameter of the artery decreases. The *embolus* sticks there and blocks the blood flow to the destination artery. The *arterial system* may be likened to the branching system of a tree. From the trunk to the periphery of the tree each branch gets smaller. If one of the branches is obstructed, the leaves supplied by that branch will starve to death. In humans, unlike the situation in trees, some brain areas receive blood from two sources. In these cases the recovery from the stroke is much better since there are alternate blood supplies. The *embolus* is usually a piece of a blood clot or *plaque* that has formed in a larger artery and broken off. The piece is then washed through the arteries and branches until it winds up at a "fork in the road" that is too small for it to pass. CranioSacral Therapy is good for these patients as soon as their condition is stabilized and they are off the critical list. Similarly, the more time that passes between the stabilization and the application of Cranio-Sacral Therapy, the less dramatically beneficial the results will be. Optimal results can be obtained if the patient begins treatment within one or two months.

The third type of stroke is the *thrombosis*. In this situation an artery closes off due to "hardening of the arteries" and/or *plaque*. This blocks blood flow, and usually an area of the brain dies. The final result depends upon the brain area that is affected.

One very dramatic case about a year ago involved a sixty-five-year-old man who had a stroke, probably due to an *embolus,* during a heart test called a *cardiac catheterization.* After the stroke he lost his ability to write by hand, and he could not put words together well enough to convey his meaning. His attempts at speech sounded like gibberish. I evaluated him about two weeks after his stroke. I located the brain area that was involved. I then mobilized his *dural membrane system,* released an *energy cyst* from the involved brain area, and did some general balancing of the *craniosacral system.* He seemed a bit dazed, which is not unusual after a CranioSacral Therapy treatment of significant depth. He got it together, with his wife's help, and the three of us walked out to the reception area together. At the reception counter, in very clear words, he asked how much he owed. He was told, and he then asked his wife for the checkbook and wrote a check. He said, "I can write again." Then he stopped after a few seconds and said, "I'm talking too." I agreed, made an appointment for him in a week, and left him and his wife to indulge their initial amazement. At the next appointment he was fine. Soon he went back to work as a salesman.

Post-Operative Rehabilitation

CranioSacral Therapy is an excellent addition to the program of rehabilitation from any kind of surgery. It restores the movement of body fluids to any areas that have been traumatized by the surgical procedures. In so doing, CranioSacral Therapy enhances the healing process and holds the potential for reducing the formation of adhesions and the extent of scarring.

I discussed previously in this book my early experiences working with a neurosurgeon on his post-operative brain-surgery patients. I recommend CranioSacral Therapy for the post-operative patient of any type of surgery, beginning about ten days to two weeks following the date of the operation. In addition to minimizing adhesion formation and excess scarring, CranioSacral Therapy will aid in removing the residual toxicity of the anesthetic and pain medications that were used. These residual toxicities often slow the recovery process for the patient. Even months or years following surgery, CranioSacral Therapy can help in the treatment of internal adhesions and excessive restrictive scars that have formed, and it can clear residual toxicities from the medications that were used. The sooner CranioSacral Therapy is begun, however, the better it is at preventing complications.

I recently treated a patient who had undergone three brain surgeries within five months. He came here from Switzerland approximately three months after his last operation. I treated this man three times per week for three weeks. During this time he recovered his energy, which may or may not have happened as a result of his treatments. He believed that Cranio-Sacral Therapy was very effective in this area because he felt the flow of energy through his head increase during each treatment and, by the end of the first week, he was highly energized. He also experienced relief from all head pain. He regained his sense of smell. His sense of balance and equilibrium returned to normal. His mind became much more clear. And his sleeping patterns normalized. This patient returned home a very happy man.

I have used CranioSacral Therapy with similar beneficial effects in terms of recovery enhancement on all types of surgical procedures, including back surgeries; *liver, heart* and *kidney transplants;* abdominal surgical procedures for a multitude of reasons; breast surgeries; *hysterectomies; Caesarean sections;* and even three cases of leg amputations. I have not yet had a post-operative patient who did not express positive feelings regarding the treatment he or she received.

6

Partial Summary of the Applications of CranioSacral Therapy

In previous parts of this text I have mentioned many of the following problems and given case histories. In brief I will summarize them for you now and mention a few that I have not described before.

Seizures. We talked a lot about *seizures.* Our success is usually good. Sometimes the situation is totally reversed—medication is no longer required and the *seizures* cease. More often, medication is still required for prevention, but the required dose is usually less than half of what was necessary before. A small number of seizure patients don't respond to CranioSacral Therapy. I have been treating *seizure* patients since 1975 and have yet to see an adverse reaction.

Learning Disabilities. I have treated a great number and variety of learning-disabled children. In my experience, over half of these children had problems with the *craniosacral system.* I feel very safe in saying that when a *craniosacral system* problem is present in a learning-disabled child and the problem is corrected, the child has a ninety percent chance of overcoming his learning disability. Most often the disability simply disappears.

Cerebral Palsy. This is a catchall term. All it means is that the brain doesn't work right. The implication that goes with the diagnosis is that the problem was present at birth. We do well with the majority of *cerebral palsy* patients. The rule holds that the sooner we can treat them the better they will do. I suspect that the initial problem the child has prevents him or her from doing certain things. If these things are not done (because they can't be done) for the first few years of life, the *nerve pathways* necessary to perform these things do not develop. If we have the honor of treating the patient as an adolescent, even if we are able to correct the original problem, the necessary *nerve pathways* may not be present. Then it becomes a question of whether, at this later date and with the problem corrected, this patient can develop the necessary nerves and circuits. The answer is probably yes, but a lot of work and training may be required.

Motor and Speech Problems. These are problems not diagnosed as *cerebral palsy.* We can almost invariably improve these problems. We had one forty-year-old patient recently who had had trouble swallowing since birth. Release of the nerves to the swallowing mechanism as they passed out of the base of the skull corrected the problem. She went home after four treatments able to chew and swallow regular food, rather than relying on fluids and purees. She also has a speech impediment, which is improving more slowly, but improving nonetheless.

Eye-Motor Problems. Sometimes, *convergent strabismus* (cross-eyedness) and other eye-movement control difficulties are due to problems that occur as the nerves to the eyes pass between the two layers of dural membrane just beneath the base of the brain. When these membranes are strained enough to interfere with the conduction of electrical impulses *via* these nerves to the eyes, the eyes do not respond to what the brain would like them to do because the messages don't get to them. A skilled CranioSacral Therapist can tell in a matter of minutes whether membrane tension is the cause of the problem. When this is the case, especially in a small child, the problem is often permanently correctable in two or three CranioSacral Therapy sessions. Corrective surgery can then often be avoided.

Endocrine Disorders. I wish to reinforce the fact that many of these problems are responsive to CranioSacral Therapy aimed at the *pituitary* and *pineal glands* in the head and the *ovaries* and *testes* in the pelvis. Also, releasing the *dural sleeves* that may be restricting nerve outflow to the *adrenals,* the *thyroid*, the *spleen*, the *liver*, and the *thymus glands* has been very helpful in some patients.

Newborns. CranioSacral Therapy seems very effective as a general health enhancer in newborns and as specific treatment for *colic, seizures, strabismus, floppy-baby syndrome, cerebral palsy,* breathing problems, and a myriad of other things. I would truly like to see CranioSacral Therapy used within forty-eight hours of delivery for each newborn. I'm sure that the incidence of brain dysfunctions could be reduced by at least fifty percent, excluding cocaine babies and genetic defects. The evaluation and treatment of newborns could effectively be carried out by nurses and by midwives in home-delivery circumstances.

Labor and Childbirth. CranioSacral Therapy can be used to enhance the strength of a normal contraction, thus shortening prolonged labor. It effectively alleviates maternal back pain and relaxes the pelvis, thus easing the stresses of the delivery process on the mother. This alleviation of stresses benefits the baby significantly in that the child is not born with a high level of stress hormones, which may be destructive to tender new tissues and organs. These hormones make excessive demands upon the baby's body.

7

How Anyone Can Use the Principles and Methods of CranioSacral Therapy

There are some very simple techniques you can use no matter what your training or background. All you have to do is trust yourself to do them. You can learn to use your hands to enhance the self-corrective and self-healing powers that we all possess. I am not suggesting that you become a "healer." The body you are working with is the healer. You are the facilitator. I believe we have all been born with more or less ability to assist the natural healing processes that are inherent in all of us.

The Upledger Institute presents a one-day hands-on workshop called ShareCare®. This workshop is for nonprofessionals and professionals alike. It simply introduces you to the experience of helping a body to balance itself and heal. You are assisting that body's self-corrective mechanisms. The body can be yours or someone else's.

We also spend a lot of time teaching parents to treat their children, especially if these children are handicapped and would benefit from ongoing CranioSacral Therapy. In these cases we like to evaluate and treat the child first with the parents present. As we develop an ongoing treatment program, we teach parents what they can do on a regular basis using the Cranio-

Sacral Therapy techniques we have taught them. This gives the family some independence from the CranioSacral Therapist, who will perhaps re-evaluate every six months or so.

There are essentially four hands-on techniques that anybody can safely apply. They are: 1) Still-Point Induction; 2) Parietal Lift Technique; 3) Decompression of the Temporomandibular Joints; and 4) Direction of Energy.

1. Still-Point Induction

In CranioSacral Therapy, a *still point* is a period lasting from several seconds to several minutes during which the activity of the *craniosacral system* is temporarily interrupted. During a *still point* it would appear that the system is reorganizing and finding ways to increase its effectiveness. When the *craniosacral rhythm* recommences after a *still point,* it is usually more powerful, more symmetrical, and feels more at ease. In other words, the hands-on observer gets a sense that the system is

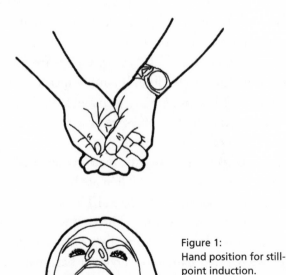

Figure 1:
Hand position for still-point induction.

not straining as much. Some of its resistances have been "dissolved."

The induction of a *still point* in a body, be it your own or another person's, is beneficial. It reduces stress. It calms the *nervous system*. It lowers blood pressure. It can reverse a fever. It increases *immune system* effectiveness. It treats headaches, arthritis, and so on. The induction of a *still point* on a daily basis is a wonderful tonic for your body.

* * *

A few years ago my own son came into the house and showed me an infected cut on his foot. I examined him and found that the *lymph channels* going up his leg to his groin were infected, and the *lymph nodes* (glands) in his groin were swollen, red and painful. His temperature was elevated to 102.5 degrees Fahrenheit. Clearly, this was an infection that was spreading and could result in serious trouble. I laid him down on the couch with his head in my hands. I induced three or four *still points* in a row. As I did, I could feel the fever in his head dropping to normal. He went to sleep. I re-examined his leg and groin about an hour later. The redness and swelling of the *lymph nodes* were gone. They were no longer tender. I could not trace the *lymph channels* up from the foot. We cleaned and put some antiseptic on the cut. That was all there was to it. His fever never returned and there was no sign of recurrence of the infection. I did *not* heal my son. I facilitated his own healing. The *still points* I induced enhanced the movement of all his body fluids, thus enabling his immune system to work more effectively.

* * *

This case concerns a good friend whose wife was suffering from severely elevated high blood pressure. The medications she was taking left her feeling "drugged" and unable to enjoy her life. She was in her mid-sixties. I showed her husband how to induce a *still point*. He had no medical training and did not feel the subtle rhythm of the *craniosacral system*. He was probably fearful of doing something wrong, so he prevented himself from feeling this subtle *craniosacral rhythm*. I taught him how to use the hand-placement technique on his wife's head. (See Figure 5.) I told him to simply let her head rest on his hands in this special way for fifteen minutes every morning. I knew that within fifteen minutes his wife would go through at least three or four *still points*. Whether he could feel the rhythm changes or not didn't matter. There is no such thing as an "overdose" of *still points*. He fearfully followed my instruction, and after a few days he gained confidence as he saw no ill effects. His fear left. His confidence went even higher as he saw her blood pressure dropping. She monitored her blood pressure daily. Soon she began to "forget" to take her medication. He continues to do the Still-Point Inductions daily. His self-esteem is improved because he feels useful. He can participate in his wife's healthcare rather than helplessly watch her deteriorate from his active, energetic wife to a dull and listless woman on medication. From her perspective, he touched her in a kind and loving way for at least fifteen minutes every morning. Their relationship grew and blossomed as he felt useful and she felt his love. This too might lower blood pressure. In either case, the *still point* is the inducer.

* * *

There have been many occasions where I have wanted still points induced on a daily basis for people who have no significant other, who travel a lot, who want to be independent and do it themselves, etc. In answer, I developed the Still-Point Inducer as a substitute method for those times when a skilled therapist isn't on-hand. The Inducer is made of two attached foam spheres covered by soft latex. To use it correctly, you simply lie down in a relaxed position on your back with the Inducer against the base of your skull for ten to twenty minutes. Used daily, it can help relieve headaches and migraines; ease chronic musculoskeletal pain; increase vitality; enhance immune system efficiency; facilitate your body's self-correcting abilities; reduce stress; and promote a sense of well-being. To order a Still-Point Inducer, call 1-800-233-5880, ext. 35556.

* * *

Actually, the *still point* can be induced from any area on the body. In response to the *craniosacral system* the whole body is continually rotating externally and internally.

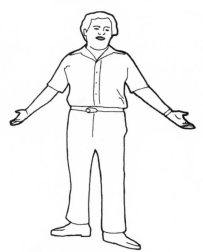 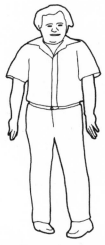

Figure 2:
Whole-body habitus of chronic craniosacral flexion.

Figure 3:
Whole-body habitus of chronic craniosacral extension.

* * *

When you hold the same body parts on both sides in internal rotation over a period of fifteen minutes, you will induce a still point. Do not apply a lot of force when working with the legs— only perhaps enough to pick up an eight-ounce glass of water. You may begin to feel the gentle internal and external rotation of these body parts. If so, just follow the rotation and hold it in its internal position. If you feel the body attempting to externally rotate, resist those attempts. When the body stops trying, the *still point* has been induced. The illustration in Figure 4 shows how the hands are placed to induce a *still point* from the feet. The same principles can be used from the calves, knees or thighs, as well as the hands, wrists, lower arms, elbows and upper arms. Use whatever body parts are most comfortable and convenient to both you and your subject. Remember, it is important to hold both sides of the body equally and in the same places.

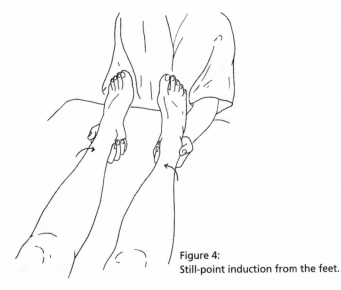

Figure 4:
Still-point induction from the feet.

The most effective place for the induction of a *still point* is the head. Your hands should be held with one hand lying over the other and the thumb tips touching so that they form a "V," as in figure 1. The backs of your hands should be be laid upon the surface of the bed, table, couch, floor, or whatever your subject is lying upon.

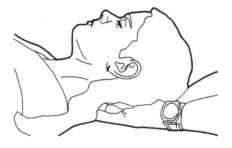

Figure 5:
Hand position for still-point induction at the head.

The back of your subject's head should rest upon your hands so that the occipital protuberance (bony protuberance) rests between your thumbs in the "V" formed by them.

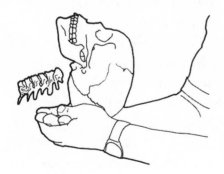

Figure 6:
Relations of hand positions to bony structures for still-point induction at the head.

The position should be comfortable for both of you. If not, do some minor positional adjusting until it is comfortable. Now all you have to do is wait in this position about fifteen minutes. Your subject will certainly experience three or four still points during this time. This is a wonderful technique.

2. The Parietal Lift

This is a technique that I have taught to hundreds of university students as well as a great many patients and laypersons. It simply involves lifting the *parietal bones,* which form a generous portion of the roof of the skull, in order to improve blood flow to the brain. For university students it is handy because they can use it on themselves to fight mental fatigue while they are sitting at their desks taking exams. For elderly citizens grappling with a little bit of memory loss or having small strokes and other symptoms due to somewhat insufficient blood supply to the brain, it is an excellent helper. It is easy to do, it takes only a few minutes, and it can be done by a significant other, a friend, or by yourself.

A seventy-six-year-old lady, whom I was caring for as a family doctor, came in to see me after falling and injuring her knee on the sidewalk. I asked her if she had tripped or slipped or stubbed her toe. None of the above was the right answer. She had experienced a momentary blackout and had fallen on the sidewalk. As we talked, she described several such "light-headed" episodes, but this was the first time she had fallen down. There are two large arteries (the carotid arteries) going from the chest up to the head. Located on the front of each side of the neck fairly close to the Adam's apple, they are reasonably accessible to an examiner's fingers. When one of these arteries is compressed by my finger pressure, there should be enough blood going through the other *carotid artery,* as well as the *vertebral arteries* in back of the neck, to compensate for the temporary reduction of blood flow caused by my finger pressure on one *carotid artery.* This pressure should not produce fainting or light-headedness if there is adequate blood supply to the brain. I pressed gently on one *carotid artery* and she almost fainted. I produced this effect no matter which side I pressed. Obviously she was not getting quite enough blood to her brain. This was the *small-stroke syndrome,* more recently called the transient *ischemic attack.* By either name it is a warning that a stroke is on the way. Her husband was eighty years of age at the time. He was in pretty good health, so I told him and his wife about the Parietal Lift Technique to increase blood flow to the brain. I told them it should be done daily in order to improve blood supply to the brain. I offered to teach him how to do it. He accepted, learned quickly, and was soon doing it on his wife daily, sometimes twice daily, he informed me. Her condition improved, she had no more small strokes, nor did she have the big one. The Parietal Lift was certainly effective for her, and her husband felt great about being a participant in her healthcare rather than just a helpless observer. They stayed in my practice for about three years after that, and then they moved up north to join their daughter and her family. I lost track of them after that.

The Parietal Lift is a two-step procedure when done by a professional; as a layperson, you will get a positive effect by doing the procedure in one step. In this way it does not require you to feel all the subtle changes that the CranioSacral Therapist learns to take for granted. All you do in the one-step procedure is place the pads of your fingers on the sides of the *parietal bones* as indicated in the illustration.

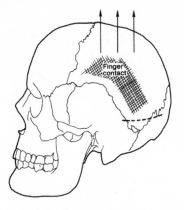

Figure 7:
Parietal Lift with traction.

Be sure that your fingers are placed above the suture joints between the *parietal bones* and the *temporal bones* on the sides. Also be sure that your fingers are placed on the *parietal bones* behind the *suture joint* between the forehead *(frontal bone)* and the *parietal bones*. You will be correct if your forwardmost finger on each side is straight up from the ear canal, and if your fingers are about two inches above the tops of the ears.

The next illustration demonstrates how your hands are placed above the head.

The thumbs are crossed above the subject's head, but not touching the head. Very gently compress the *parietal bones* medially (toward the center of the head). Now a gentle pull is exerted as though you are lifting off the top of the head. Hold this position for about two minutes, then gently and slowly release your pull and remove your hands. Done once or twice a day this will improve blood flow to the brain.

To do this on yourself place the heels of your hands on the contact points indicated in the previous illustration. Lace your fingers above your head. It is best if you are sitting at a table. Gently compress the *parietal bones* medially, then pull up for about two minutes. You will feel things change in your head. This is a very healthy technique.

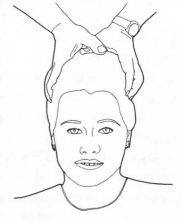

Figure 8:
Hand position for Parietal Lift.

3. Temporomandibular Joint Decompression

We discussed previously how the temporomandibular joint

has become a problem for so many people these days. Self-treatment or helping a friend or loved one suffering this problem is really quite simple. You gently pull down on the *mandible* (lower jaw), as shown in the illustration, and you will effect a decompression.

Figure 9:
Biomechanics of TMJ.

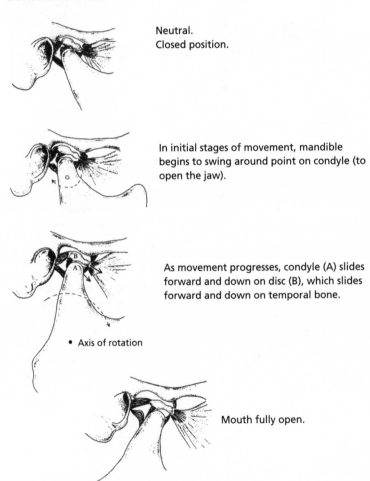

Neutral.
Closed position.

In initial stages of movement, mandible begins to swing around point on condyle (to open the jaw).

As movement progresses, condyle (A) slides forward and down on disc (B), which slides forward and down on temporal bone.

• Axis of rotation

Mouth fully open.

To do it yourself you simply pull your jaw down gently, or insert a fulcrum between your teeth, and gently push up the front of your mandible (lower jaw) as in the illustration.

Figure 10:
TMJ Disc Dysfunction.

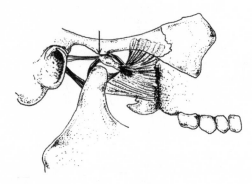

This picture shows how mandible and/or disc can "slip" past temporal eminence—"dislocation" jaw and/or "catching"disc.

Hypertonic pterygoid muscle can pull the disc forward and hold it there. Over time, this constant pull can alter the normally elastic retrodiscal tissue so that it no longer has the tendency to pull the disc back into the temporal fossa.

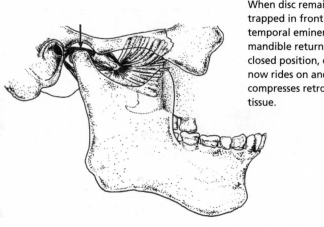

When disc remains trapped in front of temporal eminence, and mandible returns to closed position, condyle now rides on and compresses retrodiscal tissue.

Either decompression technique will work quite effectively. The trick is to use a very gentle pull if you are going straight down or a very gentle push if you are using the fulcrum technique. If you use too much force, the massive muscles of the chewing (masticatory) system will begin to resist. If you increase your force, the muscles will increase their resistance. These muscles may not relax when you give up. This could make the problem worse. Just use enough force to get a little relaxed stretch in the muscles. As soon as you feel them tighten against you, lighten up just a little so that these muscles do not feel like they are working against you. Doing it on yourself is sometimes easier than having it done by someone else; you may become aware of your own jaw tightening more readily than someone else would. Remember in this case, less is better than more. A little force over a longer time will get the job done without recruiting resistance.

4. Direction of Energy

This is a technique that anyone can learn. It is the gift that everyone is born with. It is also a gift that is perhaps most incompatible with our scientific and high-tech approaches to life in these modern times. On the other hand, the concept and techniques I shall present to you, and the results achieved, were acceptable to the biophysicists with whom I was working at the time I discovered them.

The techniques involve placing your hands on either side of a hurt area and envisioning that you are passing energy through the subject's body part from hand to hand. (See Figure 11.) You envision the energy and mentally suggest to yourself it is the kind of energy needed to help heal the tissues through which you are passing the energy. All that is required is that you accept that you can do it and that you not decide

what is needed. The qualities of the passed energy are determined by the subject's tissues. Most of the people who find
that they cannot do it are the ones who find it impossible to
believe it can happen.

In some of our experiments we created an electrical circuit
between myself and the patient. First we measured the resistance in the circuit before I touched the patient. Then we measured it after I touched the patient without applying any specific intention. Then we measured it again as I intended to put
energy into the patient, but of a certain type of my own choos-
ing. Finally we measured it as I silently asked the patient's tissues what they needed and I agreed to offer, to the best of my
ability, the quality of energy preferred by them. The results
were most remarkable. In general, before touch there were
usually over three million ohms of resistance. Typically, when
I touched with both hands the ohms dropped to about three
hundred thousand. When I put in my own intention, we would
get a typical initial drop to perhaps one hundred thousand
ohms, then a rise as it seemed that the patient's tissues realized
I was doing *my* thing and not *theirs*. By this I mean that I was
deciding what they needed rather than doing what their tissues told me. When I offered to provide just the energy that
the involved tissues wanted, the ohms would typically drop to
fifty thousand or lower. The lowest I ever achieved was about
four hundred ohms. Then we tried inserting various materials
between my hand and the patient. None of the materials we
used made any difference. They did not increase the resistance
in the circuit. The materials we tested were one-inch-thick rub-
ber, a lead shield, a two-inch piece of wood, one-inch plywood,
a one-quarter-inch-thick glass plate, a sixteen-layer-thick alu-
minum foil, and an ultraviolet filter. The only thing that
occurred was that it might have taken a few seconds for the

energy being passed to penetrate the interposed materials. Conversely, the ultraviolet filter reduced the resistance in the circuit even further. We did some more complicated work, and all of it confirmed the existence of the passage of energy.

We teach this passage of energy to children. In general, they seem quicker to pick it up and accept it than adults do. This is probably because they have not yet learned that this is "impossible."

This work can be used to aid in the reduction of pain from recent sprains, bruises, and so on. It was reported to me that a lady in extreme post-surgical pain from a leg amputation received the Direction of Energy technique through her bandages from a male nurse. He reported that she required no pain medication through the night, and throughout her hospital stay required much less than expected. I have used it thousands of times. I usually don't say what I am doing because a skeptical patient can block the effect to some extent.

Let's pretend that you have sprained your knee. All I have to do is place your knee between my two hands. I then silently intend to offer the energy that will best serve the damaged tissues. I will then feel energy begin to move towards one hand or the other. When this direction becomes clear I pretend that one hand or one finger is the sender and the other is the receiver. Then the receiving hand will probably feel heat coming out. When the energy stops flowing and the head radiation stops, we are

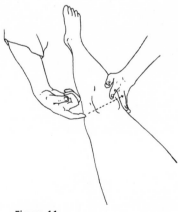

Figure 11:
Directing energy through the knee.

finished for now. Your knee will probably feel at least fifty percent better. We may repeat in a few minutes. If a similar response
occurs, we repeat the process. Repeats are done until there is
little or no perceptible response.

The Inner Physician Once Again

I have mentioned that each of us has an Inner Physician inside
that knows the answers to our health problems. When you are
inducing *still points* in a friend or loved one, they get very
relaxed. They get into an *alpha state*. This is the ideal time to
very respectfully invite the Inner Physician to come forward
and get acquainted. Many times this will happen. Just ask
whatever questions you have and wait for the answers to come
through the voice of your subject. This is fun to explore, and
once a rapport and trust are developed, you and your subject
may gain invaluable information about health problems and
how to resolve them. This requires only common sense to do.
Enjoy.

Index

Biography of John E. Upledger, DO, OMM

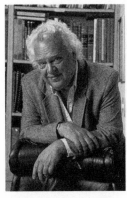

Dr. John E. Upledger is the President of The Upledger Institute, Inc. Dedicated to the natural enhancement of health, the Institute is recognized worldwide for its groundbreaking continuing-education programs, clinical research, and therapeutic services.

Throughout his career as an osteopathic physician, Dr. Upledger has been recognized as an innovator and leading proponent in the investigation of new therapies. His development of CranioSacral Therapy in particular has earned him an international reputation. He has also served on the Alternative Medicine Program Advisory Council for the Office of Alternative Medicine at the National Institutes of Health in Washington, DC.

Although much of his experience has been garnered through private clinical practice, Dr. Upledger served from 1975-1983 as a clinical researcher and Professor of Biomechanics at Michigan State University. During those years he supervised a team of anatomists, physiologists, biophysicists, and bioengineers in experiments testing the existence and influence of the craniosacral system.

The results of those scientific studies explained the function of the craniosacral system and its use in evaluating and treating poorly understood malfunctions of the brain and spinal cord. Dr. Upledger went on to develop and refine CranioSacral Therapy and other complementary modalities, which are now taught worldwide to a diverse group of healthcare professionals through The Upledger Institute's educational programs. He has also written numerous textbooks and study guides, and more than two dozen research articles.

Dr. Upledger later established The Upledger Foundation to reach out to those less fortunate to help improve their life experiences. This nonprofit organization is dedicated to the ongoing research and development of new therapeutic applications, and the establishment of community-outreach programs that enhance total health. Some of the current programs conducted by the Foundation include: performing CranioSacral Therapy techniques within the unique context of an aquatic environment in BioAquatic Exploration, increasing self-esteem in young children through the Compassionate Touch Program, and treating Post-Traumatic Stress Disorder in Vietnam veterans. For more information on these programs, please visit www.upledger.com.

Contact Information

For information on healthcare continuing-education workshops for professionals and educational materials (modalities include CranioSacral Therapy, SomatoEmotional Release®, Mechanical Link^sm, Visceral Manipulation, Lymph Drainage Therapy^sm, Therapeutic Imagery and Dialogue, and related techniques):

> The Upledger Institute, Inc.®
> 11211 Prosperity Farms Road D-325
> Palm Beach Gardens, FL 33410-3487
> Phone: 1-800-233-5880
> Fax: 561-622-4771
> Home page: www.upledger.com
> E-mail: upledger@upledger.com

For patient information on CranioSacral Therapy or clinical services:

> The Upledger Institute, Inc. HealthPlex Clinical Services
> 11211 Prosperity Farms Road D-223
> Palm Beach Gardens, FL 33410-3487
> Phone: 561-622-4706
> Fax: 561-627-9231
> Home page: www.upledger.com
> E-mail: uihealthplex@upledger.com

To Find a Practitioner

The International Association of Healthcare Practitioners® (IAHP) publishes a directory of more than 40,000 healthcare practitioners that includes their professional designations, telephone numbers, and listing of the IAHP-recognized courses they have completed. To order or for more information, call Educational Services at 1-800-311-9204, or visit www.iahp.com.